UNSTOPPABLE WOMEN EMBRACING THEIR FIRE

Kim Huynh

DEDICATION

To my beloved friends and family,

Without your love, encouragement, and steadfast support, this journey would have been impossible. You have been my shelter in the storms, my source of strength in moments of doubt, and my loudest cheerleader through every success and setback. Even when I struggled to believe in myself, your belief in me has been my greatest gift. Each of you has played an irreplaceable role in my story — whether through your words, presence, or unwavering love. I dedicate this to you, with all my heart, as a testament to the power of community, friendship, and family. Thank you for walking beside me on this incredible journey. Your unwavering love, support, and belief in me have been my greatest strength.

Through every high and low, you have been my anchor, lifting me when I stumbled and celebrating every triumph along the way. Your endless patience, wisdom, and encouragement have guided me, while your humor and kindness have lightened the load. Your courage to speak the truth, your willingness to listen, and your strength to stand beside me have shaped this journey more than words can express. This book would not exist without the generosity, resilience, and inspiration each of you has shown me. Every step of this path, every page of this book, is a testament to the love and strength you've given me. Thank you for being my biggest cheerleader, my source of inspiration, and my safe haven. This journey is as much yours as it is mine — my heart is forever grateful for each of you.

With all my heart,

Kim Huynh

UNSTOPPABLE WOMEN

ACKNOWLEDGMENTS

To every woman who has ever questioned her strength or doubted her worth, this book is for you. I want to acknowledge the fierce, unstoppable spirit within you waiting to be ignited. You are powerful beyond measure, and your fire is needed. May this book be a reminder that you can rise, thrive, and blaze your trail, no matter what the obstacles are before you. Also, who inspired me on this journey — your courage, resilience, and unapologetic passion have been the heart and soul of this work. I am deeply grateful for the stories you've shared, the wisdom you've so generously imparted, and the ways you've shown me what it truly means to embrace your fire. You have shown me that being unstoppable isn't about perfection but about perseverance and authenticity. Your influence and strength are woven into every page of this book.

To my family and friends, I cannot thank you enough for your unwavering support throughout this process. Your belief in me and this project has been my foundation. You lifted me when I was weary, cheered me on when I doubted myself, and reminded me of my purpose when the path felt uncertain. Your love, encouragement, and patience have meant more to me than words can express. Thank you for holding space for me, for allowing me to grow, and for always being the flame that reignited my spirit when it began to dim.

To my readers, thank you for picking up this book and embarking on this journey with me. Your time, attention, and energy are deeply valued. I hope that within these pages, you find the inspiration to embrace your fire and unleash your unstoppable spirit. Know that you are not alone on this journey and that together, we can create a world where women are empowered to stand in their truth and live fiercely. You also have walked with me through this process, this book reflects the collective power we hold when we come together. You have helped me not only write this book but live its message. We are all part of a powerful movement of unstoppable women, and for that, I am eternally grateful.

TABLE OF CONTENTS:

Introduction:

As I sit here, my fingers poised over the keyboard, I can't help but reflect on the journey that brought me to this point. It is a journey filled with challenges, triumphs, and a burning desire to be unstoppable. The flames of determination and resilience that have been kindled within me over the years have shaped me into the woman I am today. From an early age, I learned the power of persistence. I watched my father navigate the rough waters of life, facing countless obstacles with unwavering grace and strength. He taught me that being unstoppable was not about falling, but rising every time life knocked you down. His lesions were etched into my heart, forming the foundation of my determination.

As a young girl, I had big dreams. I envisioned myself soaring high above the clouds breaking through the barriers that looked to hold me back. The world was full of possibilities, and I was determined to explore them all. I didn't know it then, but that fiery determination that burned deeply within me would drive me forward in the face of adversity.

Growing up, I faced my fair share of challenges. Life tested my resolve time and time again. There were moments when I questioned whether I had the strength to keep moving forward, but that indomitable spirit within me never allowed me to stay down for long. It was as if there was an inner fire, burning brightly, fueling my determination to whatever obstacles lay in my path. In a world that sometimes seemed content to hold me back, I learned being unstoppable was a choice. It was a decision to keep pushing forward, even when the odds were stacked against me. It was a commitment to embracing the fire within, letting it light the way through the darkest of times.

Through the years, I have watched countless women rise

above their circumstances, breaking through the glass ceilings, and shattering the stereotypes that society imposed on them. I have seen strength, resilience, and an unyielding determination in the faces of the women who refused to be confined by the limitations others tried to impose upon them. As I look back on my journey, I am grateful for the lessons I have learned and the strength I have gained. I understand that being unstoppable is not about having all the answers or never feeling fear. It is about acknowledging the fear, and yet moving forward anyway. It is about embracing the uncertainty and boldly stepping into the unknown.

The path to becoming unstoppable is not without its challenges, but it is a journey that is worth every step. It is a journey of self-discovery, growth, and the realization that the power to be unstoppable lies within each one of us. It is a journey of breaking free from the constraints that society places on women and forging our own paths, unapologetically.

In the chapters that follow, we will explore the stories of women who have defied the odds, shattered the barriers, and risen to greatness. We will dive into the lessons they have learned, the obstacles they have overcome, and the wisdom they have gained along the way. So, as we embark on this journey, I invite you to embrace the fire within you, to be unapologetically you, and to discover the unstoppable force that lies at the core of every woman. Together, we will draft our own stories of triumph, resilience, and unwavering determination, proving that we are, indeed, unstoppable.

In the pursuit of being unstoppable, I realized that one of the most critical factors that shaped my journey was the power of belief. Belief in myself, my dreams, and the unwavering conviction that I could overcome any obstacle that crossed my path. It was this belief that ignited the flame of determination within me and kept it burning brightly through the darkest of times. Belief is a formidable force. It is the driving energy that propels us forward when the road ahead seems treacherous and uncertain. It is the catalyst for taking that first step into uncharted territory, even when our knees tremble with uncertainty. I have often heard it said that if you do not believe in yourself, no one else will, and I could not agree more.

Growing up, I was fortunate to have mentors and role models who instilled in me the belief that I could achieve anything I set my mind to. They were the guiding stars that helped me navigate the murky waters of self-doubt and hesitation. They showed me that, with an unwavering belief in my abilities, there were no limits to what I could accomplish.

Belief is not something that is simply given to us. It is something we must cultivate and nurture within ourselves. It requires looking within, acknowledging our strengths and weaknesses, and then choosing to focus on the former. It is about recognizing that every obstacle we encounter is an opportunity for growth and a chance to prove our resilience. I remember a time in my life when I faced a significant setback. It felt as if all the doors were closing, and the weight of disappointment threatened to extinguish the fire within me. But in that moment of darkness, I turned to the power of belief. I remembered the countless women who had faced adversity head-on and emerged stronger on the other side.

I reminded myself that I, too, possess the same strength, the same determination, and the same unwavering belief. With renewed conviction, I started taking small steps towards my goal, each one fueled by the belief that I could overcome the obstacles in my path. Slowly but surely, the tide began to turn, and I found myself making progress. It was a powerful lesson that reinforced the notion that, in the face of adversity, belief in ourselves is the beacon of hope that guides us through the storm.

The journey of becoming unstoppable is not a straight path. It is filled with twists and turns, moments of doubt, and challenges that evaluate the very core of our belief. But it is during these moments that we must remember that belief is not a passive force; it is an active choice. It is a decision to stand tall when the world tries to bring us down, to keep moving forward when the odds are stacked against us.

In the chapters that follow, we will explore the stories of women who harnessed the power of belief to overcome adversity, break through barriers, and achieve their dreams. We will witness how their unwavering faith in themselves, and their vision propelled them to greatness.

I invite you to reflect on the power of belief in your own life. Embrace it, nurture it, and let it fuel your journey to becoming unstoppable. Remember that you have the strength and determination to overcome any challenges that come your way, and it all begins with an unwavering belief in yourself.

1. "EMBRACING YOUR INNER STRENGTH"

EMBRACING INNER STRENGTH: A PATH TO BECOMING UNSTOPPABLE

Inner strength is a quiet but powerful force that fuels our resilience, perseverance, and authenticity. It transcends physical capability, residing in our mental and emotional fortitude, helping us overcome adversity, pursue our goals, and stay true to who we are. Recognizing and nurturing this inner strength is the first step in harnessing its transformative power.

Recognizing Your Inner Strength

1. **Self-Reflection**: Reflect on moments when you overcame difficulties. What traits helped you through—was it patience, determination, optimism? By identifying these qualities, you gain insight into your unique strengths.
2. **Mindfulness**: Cultivate mindfulness to stay aware of your thoughts and emotions. This awareness enables you to respond thoughtfully rather than react impulsively, giving you greater clarity and control.
3. **Positive Affirmations**: Reinforce your belief in yourself with daily affirmations. Remind yourself of your strengths, capabilities, and worth, building confidence and deepening your inner resilience.

The Pillars of Inner Strength: Resilience, Determination, and Compassion

Three key qualities — resilience, determination, and compassion — are the foundation of inner strength. Together, they form the core of who you are and empower you to be an unstoppable force in life.

- **Resilience**: Resilience is the ability to recover from setbacks, adapt, and keep moving forward. Life's challenges test our resolve, but it's our resilience that enables us to bend without breaking. Each time we bounce back, we reaffirm our inner strength.
- **Determination**: Determination is the unwavering commitment to achieving your goals, no matter the obstacles. It is this relentless drive that fuels progress. When you are determined, setbacks become mere steppingstones to success.
- **Compassion**: Compassion connects us to others, allowing us to empathize, support, and uplift. It is a profound strength, enabling us to foster meaningful relationships and make a positive impact on those around us.

How to Harness Your Inner Strength

1. **Set Realistic Goals**: Break large ambitions into manageable steps. Every milestone you reach enhances your confidence and reinforces your inner strength.
2. **Embrace Challenges**: Rather than seeing challenges as barriers, view them as opportunities to grow. Each obstacle you overcome adds to your reservoir of strength.
3. **Seek Support**: Surround yourself with people who uplift and encourage you. A strong support system will offer new perspectives and bolster your resolve.

4. **Cultivate Resilience**: Practice resilience by maintaining a positive outlook, learning from failures, and staying flexible in the face of change.

Real-Life Inspirations of Inner Strength

Throughout history, individuals have embodied extraordinary inner strength. Nelson Mandela, for example, endured years of imprisonment without losing his resolve, exemplifying resilience, determination, and compassion. We are surrounded by everyday heroes—people who face personal hardships with grace and resolve. These stories inspire us to tap into our inner strength.

Reflecting on Your Strength

As women, we often underestimate our inner strength. It may not be as visible as physical achievements, but it is just as powerful. By reflecting on your own experiences, you can acknowledge and embrace the qualities that make you resilient, determined, and compassionate.

1. **Resilience**: Think back to a challenging moment in your life. How did you overcome it? Your resilience is a testament to your ability to persist, adapt, and thrive. It's a reflection of your inner strength.
2. **Determination**: Recall a time when you pursued a goal with unyielding determination. What drove you forward? This determination is the force that empowers you to shape your future.
3. **Compassion**: Consider instances when you've extended compassion to others. Your empathy and kindness are profound strengths, enabling you to make a lasting difference in the lives of others.

Nurturing and Amplifying Your Inner Strength

Inner strength is not static; it grows as you do. Here are ways to nurture and harness this strength in your daily life:

1. **Cultivate Resilience**: Embrace setbacks as learning experiences. Practice self-compassion and remind yourself that challenges are a part of growth. Seek inspiration from other resilient women, and let their stories reinforce your journey.
2. **Fuel Determination**: Set clear, achievable goals and break them into manageable steps. Keep a journal or vision board to track your progress and surround yourself with a supportive community that shares your ambitions.
3. **Share Compassion**: Look for opportunities to give back to your community. Whether through volunteering, mentoring, or offering a listening ear, your compassion enriches both your life and the lives of others.

Strengthening Your Daily Practice

To make inner strength an integral part of your life, consider these practices:

- **Mindfulness and Self-Reflection**: Dedicate time daily to mindfulness or journaling. These moments of introspection help you connect with your inner strength on a deeper level.
- **Set Bold Goals**: Continue to set ambitious goals that push your boundaries. Pursuing these objectives with purpose strengthens your determination and brings fulfillment.
- **Celebrate Your Achievements**: Recognize and celebrate your victories, both big and small. This affirmation of your progress will deepen your self-belief and encourage further growth.

- **Seek Support**: Build a network of friends, mentors, and loved ones who understand and celebrate your inner strength. They will provide invaluable support when challenges arise.
- **Practice Self-Care**: Taking care of yourself—mentally, emotionally, and physically—is essential to maintaining your inner strength. Prioritize self-care and a balanced lifestyle.
- **Pay It Forward**: Use your inner strength to inspire and uplift others. By sharing your resilience, determination, and compassion, you help build a stronger, more connected community.

Embracing Inner Strength: A Path to Becoming Unstoppable

Inner strength is the invisible yet potent force within us, a source of quiet resilience, perseverance, and authenticity that fuels our ability to overcome challenges. Unlike physical prowess, inner strength resides in our mental and emotional fortitude, guiding us through adversity and propelling us toward our goals. It shapes who we are, helping us remain grounded in our values, maintain hope in tough times, and become better versions of ourselves. Recognizing and nurturing this inner strength is not only empowering but transformative, offering the foundation to live with purpose and integrity.

Recognizing Your Inner Strength

1. **Self-Reflection**: To truly understand your inner strength, begin with self-reflection. Look back at the obstacles you've overcome—whether personal, professional, or emotional. What qualities helped you prevail? Was it patience, perseverance, or optimism? By identifying the traits that carried you through difficult moments, you gain insight into your unique strengths,

allowing you to embrace and harness them more effectively.

2. **Mindfulness**: Mindfulness helps us stay present and aware of our thoughts and emotions, even in stressful situations. It enables us to approach life's challenges with calm and clarity, rather than reacting impulsively. Practicing mindfulness, whether through meditation, deep breathing, or quiet reflection, sharpens our focus and allows us to respond to adversity with intention and composure.

3. **Positive Affirmations**: Reinforcing your belief in yourself through positive affirmations can build mental resilience. Remind yourself daily of your capabilities, worth, and strength. By affirming your inner strength, you instill confidence and create a powerful mental framework that will help you weather life's storms.

The Pillars of Inner Strength: Resilience, Determination, and Compassion

Inner strength is not a singular quality — it is built on multiple core attributes. Among the most crucial are resilience, determination, and compassion. These qualities work together to create a foundation of unwavering personal strength.

- **Resilience**: Resilience is the capacity to recover from setbacks and adversity. It is the ability to bend without breaking, to rise after every fall, and to continue moving forward, no matter how difficult the journey may be. True resilience is not about avoiding pain or difficulty but learning how to adapt and grow from it. Each experience that tests our resilience also strengthens it, empowering us to handle future challenges with greater ease and confidence.
- **Determination**: Determination is the inner fire that drives us toward our goals, no matter how tough the path may become. It is the fuel that keeps us moving

forward when the road is filled with obstacles and the strength that compels us to persevere when others quit. Those with determination are guided by a clear sense of purpose, and they refuse to let setbacks derail them. Determination is not just about achieving success; it's about embracing the process of growth and relentless pursuit of improvement.

- **Compassion**: Compassion is often overlooked as a source of strength, but it plays an essential role in building inner resilience. Compassion allows us to connect deeply with others, fostering empathy and understanding. It also strengthens our emotional intelligence, helping us navigate difficult situations with kindness and care. The act of extending compassion, whether to others or us, is empowering—it reminds us that our strength is not just about personal triumph, but also about lifting those around us and making a meaningful difference in their lives.

Harnessing Your Inner Strength

Knowing that resilience, determination, and compassion form the pillars of inner strength is only the beginning. The next step is to actively harness and cultivate these qualities in your life. Here are several ways to do so:

1. **Set Realistic Goals**: Achieving a grand vision or goal can feel daunting, but by breaking it down into smaller, more manageable steps, you make progress more attainable. Each milestone you reach reinforces your confidence and bolsters your inner strength, proving to yourself that you are capable of handling challenges and reaching your dreams.

2. **Embrace Challenges**: Adversity is an inevitable part of life, but how you respond to it is what matters. Rather than avoiding challenges, embrace them as opportunities to learn, grow, and build your resilience.

Each challenge overcomes your reservoir of inner strength, and with each success, your confidence grows.

3. **Seek Support**: Surrounding yourself with supportive individuals who believe in your potential is critical. Whether friends, family, or mentors, those who uplift and encourage you during tough times offer new perspectives and give you the motivation to persevere. A strong support network can help you tap into your inner strength more effectively and remind you that you are never alone in your struggles.

4. **Practice Resilience**: Resilience is not a trait you are born with—it's a skill you cultivate. Develop it by maintaining a positive outlook even in the face of hardship. Learn from your failures and remain adaptable to change. The more resilient you become, the more easily you will bounce back from life's inevitable setbacks.

Real-Life Inspirations of Inner Strength

When we look at history and everyday life, we find countless examples of inner strength. Nelson Mandela, who spent 27 years in prison and emerged with a message of peace and reconciliation, embodied resilience, determination, and compassion. His story serves as a reminder of the power of the human spirit to overcome even the most profound adversity.

Closer to home, we encounter everyday heroes who demonstrate inner strength in quieter ways. Mothers who sacrifice for their families, professionals who rise after career setbacks, or individuals who conquer personal struggles—these stories are all testaments to the extraordinary capacity of human resilience and determination.

Reflecting on Your Strength

It's important to take time to acknowledge your inner strength. Too often, we overlook our resilience, determination, and compassion, but these qualities are the cornerstone of our ability to succeed and thrive in life.

1. **Resilience**: Reflect on a challenging situation in your life. How did you navigate it, and what did you learn from the experience? Acknowledge your ability to endure and adapt—your resilience is a source of power that will continue to grow with every challenge you face.
2. **Determination**: Think of a time when you set a goal and pursued it with unshakable resolve. What gave you the strength to continue even when the path was difficult? Your determination to achieve your goals is a profound aspect of your inner strength, reminding you that you have the power to shape your future.
3. **Compassion**: Compassion is often a reflection of our deeper emotional strength. Think about moments when you have shown kindness and empathy to others, even when it was difficult. This emotional capacity is not only a strength for yourself but a gift you give to the world, fostering deeper connections and contributing to a more compassionate society.

Nurturing and Amplifying Your Inner Strength

Your inner strength is not fixed; it evolves as you do. By continually nurturing it, you ensure it becomes a reliable source of power throughout your life. Here's how to amplify it further:

1. **Mindfulness and Self-Reflection**: Make it a habit to practice mindfulness or engage in self-reflection each day. Taking moments to assess your thoughts,

emotions, and challenges allows you to connect more deeply with your inner strength and develop greater emotional resilience.

2. **Set Bold Goals**: Challenge yourself to set ambitious, meaningful goals that ignite your passion and push you beyond your comfort zone. Pursuing these goals will strengthen your determination and provide a sense of purpose that keeps you motivated.

3. **Celebrate Your Achievements**: Acknowledge and celebrate each victory, no matter how small. Recognizing your accomplishments reinforces your belief in your abilities and reminds you that you are capable of achieving great things.

4. **Seek Inspiration**: Surround yourself with stories and individuals who inspire you. Learning from the experiences of other resilient, determined, and compassionate people will not only encourage you but offer valuable lessons you can apply in your journey.

5. **Pay It Forward**: Sharing your inner strength with others is one of the most powerful ways to amplify it. Be there for those who need support, whether by offering empathy, encouragement, or a helping hand. By lifting others, you amplify your strength and create a positive impact in the world.

Reflection Questions

1. Self-Assessment: Reflect on a recent challenge you faced. What qualities did you rely on to overcome it? How did your inner strength manifest during this time?

2. Personal Growth: Identify a specific moment in your life when you demonstrated resilience. How did this experience shape your understanding of your inner strength?

3. Determination: Think about a goal you are currently pursuing or one you have recently achieved. What motivated you to stay committed, and how did your determination play a role in your success?

4. Compassion: Consider a time when you showed compassion to someone else. How did this act impact your relationship with that person and how did it reinforce your inner strength?

Application Questions

1. Setting Goals: What are some realistic goals you can set for yourself that align with your current aspirations? Break these goals down into smaller steps and identify how achieving them will bolster your inner strength.

2. Embracing Challenges: How can you reframe a current or upcoming challenge as an opportunity for growth? What strategies can you use to approach it with a mindset of resilience?

3. Building Support: Who are the key individuals in your life who support and encourage you? How can you strengthen these relationships to create a more supportive network?

4. Practicing Mindfulness: How can you incorporate mindfulness into your daily routine? What specific practices (such as meditation, journaling, or quiet reflection) could help you connect more deeply with your inner strength?

Inspirational Questions

1. Role Models: Who is someone you admire for their inner strength, and what specific qualities do they possess that you would like to emulate? How can you integrate these qualities into your own life?

2. Celebrating Achievements: How can you celebrate your achievements, both big and small, to reinforce your belief in your inner strength? What methods of recognition and celebration resonate most with you?

3. Paying It Forward: In what ways can you use your inner strength to support others in their journeys? How might acts of compassion and encouragement enrich your sense of purpose and fulfillment?

Unleashing Your Inner Strength

Embracing your inner strength is more than a concept—it's a transformative journey that unfolds as you delve into self-discovery and personal growth. This chapter has explored the essential qualities that form the foundation of inner strength: resilience, determination, and compassion. By recognizing and nurturing these attributes, you equip yourself to navigate life's challenges with grace and confidence.

Resilience empowers you to adapt and persevere through adversity, turning setbacks into opportunities for growth. **Determination** fuels your pursuit of goals, driving you to overcome obstacles and stay committed to your aspirations. **Compassion** connects you to others, allowing you to build meaningful relationships and make a positive impact on the world.

As you continue to explore and strengthen these qualities, remember that inner strength is a dynamic and evolving force. It grows with your experiences, deepens with each challenge you face, and shapes your journey toward becoming the unstoppable person you aspire to be.

Key Takeaways:

1. **Resilience**: Embrace setbacks as valuable lessons and opportunities for growth. Your ability to bounce back from adversity is a testament to your inner strength.
2. **Determination**: Set clear, achievable goals and break them into manageable steps. Your unwavering commitment to these goals will propel you forward, even when faced with difficulties.
3. **Compassion**: Extend kindness and empathy to others, and also practice self-compassion. This balance enriches your relationships and enhances your emotional well-being.
4. **Self-Reflection and Mindfulness**: Regularly engage in self-reflection and mindfulness practices to deepen your connection with your inner strength and maintain clarity in your journey.
5. **Support and Inspiration**: Build a network of supportive individuals and seek out sources of inspiration. These connections and stories will reinforce your resolve and provide motivation.

As you move forward, let these insights guide you in nurturing your inner strength. Celebrate your progress, embrace challenges as growth opportunities, and continually seek ways to apply what you've learned. Your inner strength is a powerful ally, ready to support you in achieving your dreams and making a meaningful difference in the world.

Your journey toward self-discovery and empowerment is ongoing. By continually engaging with these principles and practices, you'll unlock the full potential of your inner strength and inspire others along the way. Embrace this journey with courage and commitment, and let your inner strength be the driving force behind a life of purpose, resilience, and fulfillment.

2-THE POWER OF SELF-LOVE"

The Power of Self-Love: Unlocking Your Inner Fire

Self-love is the root from which the seeds of resilience, strength, and transformation grow. It is the fuel that ignites your inner fire, the core element that allows you to harness your power, and the essence of what makes you unstoppable. For women embracing their fire, self-love is not a luxury, nor is it something to be earned; it is the source of energy that propels you forward through adversity, lights your path in darkness, and gives you the courage to rise again every time life knocks you down.

The journey to becoming an unstoppable woman begins with the choice to love yourself—deeply, radically, and unapologetically. The fire within you, that fierce, passionate energy burning in your soul, is nurtured, and sustained by self-love. But this isn't the self-love that is trivialized as bubble baths and spa days (though those moments of self-care are important); this is a deeper, more profound love—one that sees your flaws and imperfections and celebrates them as part of your unique brilliance.

The Power of Self-Love: Unlocking Your Inner Fire

Self-love is the foundation from which resilience, strength, and transformation flourish. It is the fuel that ignites your inner fire, empowering you to tap into your fullest potential and unleashing a force that makes you unstoppable. For women who dare to embrace their fire, self-love is not a luxury or a reward to be earned; it is the vital energy that propels you through adversity, lights your path during times of uncertainty, and gives you the courage to rise again after every setback.

The journey to becoming an unstoppable woman begins with the choice to love yourself — deeply, radically, and unapologetically. This love is not the shallow kind that is often equated with pampering or indulgence. While self-care is important, true self-love is about embracing all of who you are — your strengths, your flaws, your triumphs, and your scars. It is recognizing that your worth is intrinsic, and it is the foundation upon which true empowerment is built.

Embracing Your Wholeness

To fully step into your power, you must embrace your wholeness — every aspect of who you are. Self-love requires you to honor the strong and fierce parts of yourself, as well as the vulnerable, uncertain, and sometimes fearful sides. You are not defined solely by your accomplishments or the image you project to the world. You are your dreams, your struggles, and your imperfections. By accepting your wholeness, you liberate yourself from the need for external validation — you know your worth.

This profound self-acceptance fosters inner security, allowing you to move through life with quiet confidence. It empowers you to set boundaries, prioritize your well-being, and protect your energy. You become unstoppable, not because you're flawless, but because you are whole.

The Fire of Self-Love

For a woman who has embraced her fire, self-love fuels the flames of passion, creativity, and ambition. It reminds you that you deserve space in a world that often tries to make you smaller. It tells you that you are worthy of success, of every dream you hold close, and of every opportunity that comes your way. Self-love does not allow you to dim your light for the comfort of others; instead, it demands that you shine brightly and let the world adjust to your brilliance.

Self-love emboldens you to take risks, follow your instincts, and chase your wildest dreams. It empowers you to walk away from relationships or situations that do not honor your value, knowing that you deserve better. When self-doubt creeps in, self-love is the balm that reminds you that you are more than enough—always.

Breaking Free from Fear

One of the most profound powers of self-love is its ability to free you from fear. Fear of failure, fear of judgment, and fear of not being good enough often hold women back. But when you are grounded in self-love, these fears lose their grip. You no longer strive for perfection; instead, you aim for authenticity. You no longer need to please everyone; you simply honor yourself.

Self-love teaches you that failure is not the end—it is a steppingstone on your path to growth and success. When your worth is not tied to external achievements, you can take bold steps, knowing that even if things don't go as planned, you will rise again stronger and wiser. This is the essence of being unstoppable: the ability to continually rise because your fire burns from within.

Creating a Life of Purpose

When self-love becomes your foundation, everything shifts. You begin to make empowered choices, aligning your life with your deepest desires and values. You stop chasing external validation and instead cultivate inner peace. Your relationships, career, and passions begin to reflect who you truly are. With self-love guiding you, you create a life of purpose and meaning.

An unstoppable woman knows that her fire is meant to light up the world. She understands that her unique gifts and vision are meant to make an impact. To do this, she first nurtures her inner flame, ensuring it burns bright, because only then can she inspire others and live a life of fulfillment.

Owning Your Power

Self-love is the gateway to owning your power. It allows you to break free from the limitations imposed by others and societal expectations. You are defined by your truth, your values, and your dreams—not by your past or the judgments of others. When you own your power, you become unstoppable—not because you have all the answers, but because you trust yourself to figure it out along the way. You know you have the strength, resilience, and fire to overcome any obstacle and to create the life you deserve.

You are an unstoppable woman because you have chosen to love yourself fiercely. You have chosen to embrace your fire and let it guide you toward a life of purpose, passion, and power. Self-love is your armor and your light—your strength and your freedom. And with it, you are truly unstoppable.

The Transformative Journey of Self-Love

In a world that often tells us to prioritize others and to meet external expectations, self-love is a radical act of transformation. It is not selfish; it is essential to your mental and emotional well-being. Self-love is the compass that guides you toward self-acceptance, resilience, and the unwavering belief in your worth.

For many years, I walked a path where self-love seemed distant—a destination I couldn't quite reach. I prioritized the needs and opinions of others over my own, constantly seeking validation. Each step on that self-sacrificing journey left me more disconnected from myself, until I realized that the absence of self-love was holding me back from living authentically.

Embracing self-love was a turning point. It liberated me from self-doubt, guilt, and the fear of judgment. It taught me that I deserved love, care, and respect—not just from others, but from myself. The power of self-love is in its ability to heal—to forgive yourself, release regret, and embrace imperfection. It is the declaration that you are enough, just as you are.

Lessons Learned on the Journey to Self-Love

1. **Embrace Your Flaws**: True self-love begins with accepting your imperfections. Instead of hiding them, celebrate your uniqueness and recognize that your quirks make you who you are.
2. **Set Boundaries**: Self-love means respecting your boundaries. Prioritize your well-being and preserve your energy by learning to say no without guilt.
3. **Practice Self-Compassion**: Replace self-criticism with self-compassion. Treat yourself with the same kindness you would offer a friend.
4. **Let Go of Comparison**: Comparison is the enemy of self-love. Focus on your journey, celebrate your progress, and honor your unique strengths.
5. **Prioritize Self-Care**: Taking care of yourself physically, emotionally, and mentally is a vital part of self-love. Make space for activities that bring you joy and peace.
6. **Celebrate Your Achievements**: Acknowledge your victories, no matter how small. Celebrating your accomplishments reinforces your self-worth.
7. **Seek Support**: The journey of self-love can be challenging. Seek support from friends, family, or a therapist when needed.

The Power of Self-Love

Self-love is the fertile ground from which resilience, strength, and transformation blossom. It is the fuel that kindles your inner fire, the core force that enables you to tap into your innate power, and the essence that makes you unstoppable. For women embracing their inner flame, self-love is not an indulgence, nor a reward to be earned after accomplishment—it is the vital energy source that propels you through adversity, illuminates your path through darkness, and gives you the courage to rise after every fall.

The journey toward becoming an unstoppable woman begins with a deliberate choice: to love yourself—deeply, radically, and without apology. This fire within you, this fierce, passionate energy that simmers in your soul, is sustained and nurtured by self-love. But understand—this is not the kind of self-love that is trivialized through commercialized notions of pampering and spa days, although such moments of self-care have their place. This is profound. It is the love that sees your flaws, embraces your imperfections, and celebrates your unique brilliance.

Embracing Your Wholeness

To step fully into your power, you must first embrace your wholeness—every facet of your being. This means loving not only the parts of you that are strong and confident, but also the parts that are vulnerable, afraid, and uncertain. You are not merely your achievements or the polished persona you present to the world. You are the sum of your insecurities, your mistakes, your scars, and the dreams you guard deep within your heart. Embracing your wholeness is the realization that you are enough just as you are—without needing to prove anything to anyone.

This kind of love fosters a profound inner security. It liberates you from the constant need for external validation because your value becomes an intrinsic truth. You walk with quiet confidence, not because you have it all figured out, but because you trust yourself. This inner assurance is your superpower. It allows you to set boundaries without guilt, protect your energy, and prioritize your well-being. This unwavering self-assuredness becomes the bedrock of your unstoppable nature.

The Fire of Self-Love

For the woman who has claimed her fire, self-love fans the flames of passion, creativity, and ambition. It's the force that reminds you to take up space in a world that often tries to make women small. It is the conviction that you are worthy of every opportunity, every dream, and every ounce of success you seek. Self-love demands that you stop dimming your light to fit into the narrow boxes' others create for you. Instead, you blaze with unapologetic brilliance, compelling others to adjust to your glow.

This love empowers you to take risks, to trust your instincts, and to chase your boldest ambitions. It whispers, "You can do this," when doubt creeps in or when the world attempts to stand in your way. It gives you the courage to walk away from relationships, environments, and circumstances that do not honor your worth. Self-love is the balm that soothes your spirit when fear and doubt arise, constantly reminding you that you are more than enough.

The Ripple Effect of Self-Love

Self-love is not a solitary act; it creates a ripple effect that extends far beyond yourself. When you love and accept yourself, you inspire others to do the same. You become a beacon of empowerment for those around you — friends, family, colleagues—who witness your transformation from self-doubt to self-assuredness and realize that they, too, can rise.

In your relationships, self-love becomes the foundation of mutual respect and healthy boundaries. You set the standard for how others should treat you, and in doing so, you uplift the dynamic, encouraging others to reflect on their own journey of self-love. In this way, self-love is not just a personal journey but a force that heals and strengthens your connections with the world.

Self-love also compels you to advocate for change. When you understand your worth, you naturally become a voice for others who may still be searching for their power. Whether through mentoring, supporting causes that uplift others, or simply living authentically, your example encourages a collective movement toward greater self-esteem and empowerment.

Reflective Questions

1. **Personal Connection**: How do you currently practice self-love in your life? Can you identify specific actions or habits that reflect this practice?
2. **Embracing Wholeness**: What aspects of yourself do you find most challenging to embrace? How might acknowledging and celebrating these aspects contribute to your sense of wholeness?
3. **Inner Security**: How does external validation influence your decisions or self-perception? What changes can you make to shift your focus towards internal validation?
4. **Fanning Your Flames**: In what areas of your life do you feel your inner fire is burning brightest? How can you nurture these areas further to maintain and amplify your passion and creativity?

5. **Breaking Free from Fear**: What fears are currently holding you back from pursuing your goals or dreams? How might self-love help you address and overcome these fears?

6. **Purposeful Choices**: Reflect on a recent decision you made. Did it align with your values and desires, or was it influenced by external expectations? How can you ensure your future choices are more aligned with your true self?

7. **Owning Your Power**: What does owning your power mean to you personally? Can you identify any recent situations where you either stepped into or shied away from your power?

8. **Ripple Effect**: How has your journey of self-love influenced those around you? Are there specific examples of how your self-love has inspired or impacted others in your life?

Actionable Steps

1. **Self-Love Inventory**: Create a list of ways you can practice self-love daily. Include both big and small actions and commit to integrating at least one new practice into your routine each week.

2. **Boundary Setting**: Identify an area in your life where you struggle with setting boundaries. What steps can you take to establish and maintain healthy boundaries in this area?

3. **Fear Assessment**: Write down the top three fears that are currently impacting your life. For each fear, outline a plan of action on how you can address it through self-love and resilience.

4. **Purposeful Planning**: Choose one goal or dream you have been hesitant to pursue. Develop a plan that includes self-love practices to support you in taking the first step toward this goal.

5. **Support Network**: Reach out to a friend or mentor who embodies self-love. Discuss your journey and seek their advice on how to continue growing in your practice of self-love.
6. **Celebrate Achievements**: Take time to acknowledge and celebrate a recent achievement, no matter how small. Reflect on how this success reflects your self-love and personal growth.
7. **Inclusivity Practice**: Consider ways you can promote inclusivity and support others in their journey of self-love. This could involve participating in community initiatives, offering mentorship, or simply being a supportive friend.

Discussion Prompts

1. **Community Sharing**: How can we create a community that supports and encourages self-love among women? What initiatives or activities would be effective in fostering this environment?
2. **Mentorship**: How can sharing your journey of self-love with others act as a form of mentorship? What are some ways you can effectively offer guidance and support to those at the beginning of their self-love journey?
3. **Cultural Change**: In what ways can we challenge and change societal expectations that hinder self-love and empowerment for women? How can we collectively contribute to a culture that embraces and celebrates self-love?
4. **Empowerment Beyond Self**: How can the empowerment gained from self-love be used to advocate for broader social or cultural changes? What causes or movements resonate with you where your self-love journey could make a difference?

The Ripple Effect of Self-Love

It's essential to reflect on the profound insights and actionable steps we've explored. Self-love is more than a concept; it is the cornerstone of resilience, strength, and personal transformation. It ignites your inner fire, allowing you to embrace your wholeness, face fears, and pursue your passions with unwavering confidence.

We have journeyed through the essence of self-love—understanding that it is not a luxury but a fundamental right. It is the powerful force that fuels your inner brilliance, enabling you to stand tall in the face of adversity and seize the life you deserve. By embracing your imperfections, setting boundaries, and nurturing your unique qualities, you create a solid foundation for a life filled with purpose and joy.

Key takeaways from this chapter include:

1. **Embracing Wholeness**: Accept and celebrate every aspect of who you are. Your flaws and strengths, successes and setbacks—all contribute to your unique brilliance.
2. **Building Inner Security**: Shift your focus from external validation to internal confidence. Recognize your value and walk through the world with quiet self-assurance.
3. **Fanning the Flames**: Let self-love stoke the fires of passion and creativity. Pursue your dreams fearlessly and let your inner light shine brightly.
4. **Overcoming Fear**: Use self-love to confront and dismantle the fears that hold you back. Understand that failure is a steppingstone, not a barrier.
5. **Creating Purpose**: Align your choices with your deepest values and desires. Build a life that reflects who you are and what you truly want.
6. **Ripple Effect**: Recognize the broader impact of your self-love. Your journey can inspire and uplift others,

contributing to a more compassionate and empowered world.

As you continue on your path of self-discovery, remember that self-love is not a destination but a lifelong journey. It requires ongoing reflection, commitment, and self-compassion. Embrace this journey with an open heart and a willingness to grow, knowing that each step forward brings you closer to living a life of authenticity, fulfillment, and empowerment.

Continue to nurture your self-love and let it guide you as you explore new facets of yourself. Celebrate your progress, no matter how small, and remain steadfast in your pursuit of a life aligned with your true self. Your journey is a testament to the power of self-love—a force that not only transforms you but also has the potential to inspire and elevate those around you.

So, step forward with confidence and courage. Embrace your inner fire, cherish your unique journey, and remember that through self-love, you are not only becoming unstoppable but also creating a ripple of positivity and empowerment in the world.

3. CULTIVATING RESILIENCE

A Journey of Strength and Empowerment

Resilience is the quality that defines a woman's strength, endurance, and inner fortitude. It is the invisible force that enables us to rise from adversity, bounce back from life's challenges, and emerge stronger than before. Looking back on my journey, I recognize countless moments when resilience wasn't merely a choice—it was a lifeline, guiding me through my most difficult times.

Resilience is not an innate trait, but a skill that can be cultivated and refined. It is born from facing hardship, learning from it, and using those experiences to build inner strength. It is the art of bending without breaking, adapting to change, and finding opportunity in adversity.

My journey to cultivating resilience began with the understanding that life is unpredictable. It is a path marked by highs and lows, and how we respond to those lows shapes our character. I learned to embrace challenges as opportunities for growth, realizing that our true strength often reveals itself during the most difficult times.

Here are some key lessons I've learned about building resilience:

1. **Acceptance of Change**: Resilience starts with accepting that change is a constant in life. It is about acknowledging that circumstances may shift unexpectedly and adapting to thrive in new environments.

2. **Mental Toughness**: Cultivating resilience requires developing mental toughness. This means training the mind to remain strong, focused, and solution-oriented in the face of adversity, rather than becoming overwhelmed.

3. **Seeking Support**: Being resilient doesn't mean going it alone. It means recognizing when to reach out for help—whether from friends, family, or professionals. Seeking support is a sign of strength, not weakness.

4. **Embracing Failure**: Resilience is closely tied to how we view failure. It's not a dead-end but a steppingstone to success. What matters most is not falling but getting back up, time and again.

5. **Learning from Setbacks**: Every setback is an opportunity for growth. Resilience means examining the lessons hidden within our challenges and using them to strengthen our future selves.

6. **Adaptability**: Resilient women are adaptable. Rigidity can be a hindrance, and flexibility and open-mindedness are essential for navigating the twists and turns of life.

7. **Building a Support System**: Having a network of people who uplift, inspire, and encourage you is crucial. This community of support strengthens your resilience during tough times.

8. **Positive Self-Talk**: Maintaining a positive and compassionate inner dialogue is essential to resilience. Being kind to yourself in moments of adversity fosters the strength to persevere.

Resilience is not a destination but an ongoing practice of self-awareness, compassion, and the belief that you have the strength to overcome life's challenges. In the chapters ahead, we'll explore stories of remarkable women who have built resilience in their own lives. Their wisdom will remind us that resilience is a skill that can be honed, and the strength to face life's trials resides within each of us, waiting to be nurtured.

Nurturing Resilience: Practical Steps for Inner Strength

Cultivating resilience is a profound journey of discovering your inner strength. It is a process that deepens your ability to face adversity and come out stronger. Here are some practical steps to help you on your journey of resilience:

1. **Self-Reflection**: Resilience begins with self-reflection. Take time to understand your strengths, weaknesses, and triggers. Knowing yourself is the foundation on which resilience is built.
2. **Mindfulness**: Practices like meditation and deep breathing help you stay present and manage stress in challenging times. Mindfulness reduces anxiety and fosters emotional resilience.
3. **Positive Mindset**: Cultivate a positive mindset by practicing gratitude and reframing negative thoughts. Focus on growth and opportunity, even in adversity.
4. **Seek Inspiration**: Draw strength from resilient women who have faced and overcome significant challenges. Their stories can offer valuable guidance and motivation for your journey.
5. **Set Realistic Goals**: Break down big challenges into smaller, achievable steps. Setting manageable milestones can make the path forward feel less daunting.
6. **Embrace Change**: Resilience is linked to adaptability. Be flexible when circumstances shift and recognize that change often brings new opportunities.
7. **Healthy Lifestyle**: Prioritize your physical well-being. Proper nutrition, exercise, and sleep strengthen not just your body but your emotional resilience as well.
8. **Self-Care**: Engage in activities that replenish your energy, such as reading, being in nature, or pursuing a creative hobby. Self-care is essential to building resilience.

9. **Build a Support System**: Surround yourself with a network of people who provide encouragement and guidance during tough times.
10. **Learn from Setbacks**: Each setback offers a lesson. Instead of dwelling on past failures, use them as steppingstones to future success.
11. **Celebrate Small Wins**: Recognize and celebrate every achievement, no matter how small. Each victory strengthens your resilience and builds confidence.
12. **Practice Self-Compassion**: Treat yourself with kindness, especially in moments of self-doubt. Self-compassion is a cornerstone of resilience, helping you navigate challenges with grace.

Resilience is a journey of self-discovery and strength. It is about reaching within and using available resources to overcome adversity. As you cultivate resilience, you'll find that what once seemed insurmountable becomes an opportunity for growth and transformation.

Transformative Power of Resilience

Resilience is not just about survival; it is a catalyst for personal growth and transformation. It allows us to approach life with renewed strength, confidence, and fearlessness. Here's how resilience can transform you:

1. **Confidence and Empowerment**: As you nurture resilience, you become more confident in your ability to face adversity, turning challenges into steppingstones for growth.
2. **Fearlessness**: Resilience fosters fearlessness. The ability to confront setbacks with courage becomes an integral part of your character.
3. **Adaptability**: Resilient individuals are adaptable, better equipped to navigate life's unpredictable changes, and more open to new opportunities.

4. **Mental Toughness**: Resilience builds mental toughness, allowing you to remain calm, composed, and clear-headed in difficult situations.
5. **Overcoming Fear of Failure**: Resilience helps you view failure as a learning experience rather than an endpoint. You become more willing to take risks and learn from them.
6. **Enhanced Critical Thinking**: Resilient individuals are effective problem solvers, viewing challenges as opportunities for creative solutions.
7. **Deeper Self-Understanding**: Resilience allows you to discover hidden strengths, confront weaknesses, and build a more profound connection with yourself.
8. **Fulfillment and Satisfaction**: Resilient people experience a deeper sense of fulfillment, appreciating their accomplishments and valuing the journey.
9. **Compassion**: Resilience nurtures compassion—for yourself and others—allowing you to offer support and encouragement to those facing challenges.
10. **Positive Influence**: As you transform through resilience, you become a source of inspiration for those around you, motivating them to face their challenges with courage and resilience.

Resilience isn't just a defense mechanism; it's the key to unlocking personal growth, empowerment, and fearlessness. It reminds us that even in the face of adversity, we have the power to shape our destinies and become the strong, resilient women we aspire to be.

Inspiring Resilience in Others

Your journey of resilience has the power to inspire and empower those around you. Here are ways you can lead others on their paths to resilience:

1. **Lead by Example**: Demonstrating resilience through your own actions is the most powerful way to inspire others. Show them what strength looks like in the face of adversity.
2. **Storytelling**: Sharing your story can offer hope and guidance to others. By speaking openly about your challenges, you help others see that they too can overcome their obstacles.
3. **Mentoring**: Become a mentor to someone on their resilience journey. Your wisdom and insights can guide them through their challenges.
4. **Creating Safe Spaces**: Foster environments where people can explore their vulnerabilities and build resilience without fear of judgment.
5. **Promoting Inclusivity**: Resilience is for everyone. Recognize and celebrate the unique paths each person takes on their resilience journey.
6. **Supporting Causes**: By contributing to organizations that focus on empowerment and resilience, you help strengthen the collective journey of countless individuals.
7. **Lending a Helping Hand**: Offering support during someone else's challenging time can be a powerful testament to the strength of community and compassion.
8. **Amplifying Voices**: Share the stories of others who have demonstrated resilience, helping to highlight their strength and inspire a broader audience.
9. **Fostering Empathy**: Promote empathy for yourself and others, creating a compassionate environment that nurtures resilience.
10. **Advocating for Change**: Support changes in societal attitudes and systems that hinder resilience. Advocate for communities that are more inclusive, empathetic, and supportive.

By nurturing your resilience and sharing your journey, you become a beacon of hope and strength for others. Together, we can build a resilient community where each member is empowered to face adversity with courage and determination.

Cultivating Resilience: A Journey of Strength and Empowerment

Resilience is the quality that defines a woman's strength, endurance, and inner fortitude. It is the invisible force that enables us to rise from adversity, bounce back from life's challenges, and emerge stronger than before. Looking back on my journey, I recognize countless moments when resilience wasn't merely a choice—it was a lifeline, guiding me through my most difficult times.

Resilience is not an innate trait, but a skill that can be cultivated and refined. It is born from facing hardship, learning from it, and using those experiences to build inner strength. It is the art of bending without breaking, adapting to change, and finding opportunity in adversity.

My journey to cultivating resilience began with the understanding that life is unpredictable. It is a path marked by highs and lows, and how we respond to those lows shapes our character. I learned to embrace challenges as opportunities for growth, realizing that our true strength often reveals itself during the most difficult times.

Key lessons I've learned about building resilience:

1. **Acceptance of Change**: Resilience starts with accepting that change is a constant in life. It is about acknowledging that circumstances may shift unexpectedly and adapting to thrive in new environments.

2. **Mental Toughness**: Cultivating resilience requires developing mental toughness. This means training the mind to remain strong, focused, and solution-oriented in the face of adversity, rather than becoming overwhelmed.

3. **Seeking Support**: Being resilient doesn't mean going it alone. It means recognizing when to reach out for help—whether from friends, family, or professionals. Seeking support is a sign of strength, not weakness.

4. **Embracing Failure**: Resilience is closely tied to how we view failure. It's not a dead-end but a steppingstone to success. What matters most is not falling but getting back up, time and again.

5. **Learning from Setbacks**: Every setback is an opportunity for growth. Resilience means examining the lessons hidden within our challenges and using them to strengthen our future selves.

6. **Adaptability**: Resilient women are adaptable. Rigidity can be a hindrance, and flexibility and open-mindedness are essential for navigating the twists and turns of life.

7. **Building a Support System**: Having a network of people who uplift, inspire, and encourage you is crucial. This community of support strengthens your resilience during tough times.

8. **Positive Self-Talk**: Maintaining a positive and compassionate inner dialogue is essential to resilience. Being kind to yourself in moments of adversity fosters the strength to persevere.

Resilience is not a destination but an ongoing practice of self-awareness, compassion, and the belief that you have the strength to overcome life's challenges. In the chapters ahead, we'll explore stories of remarkable women who have built resilience in their own lives. Their wisdom will remind us that resilience is a skill that can be honed, and the strength to face life's trials resides within each of us, waiting to be nurtured.

Practical Steps for Inner Strength

Cultivating resilience is a profound journey of discovering your inner strength. It is a process that deepens your ability to face adversity and come out stronger. Here are some practical steps to help you on your journey of resilience:

1. **Self-Reflection**: Resilience begins with self-reflection. Take time to understand your strengths, weaknesses, and triggers. Knowing yourself is the foundation on which resilience is built.
2. **Mindfulness**: Practices like meditation and deep breathing help you stay present and manage stress in challenging times. Mindfulness reduces anxiety and fosters emotional resilience.
3. **Positive Mindset**: Cultivate a positive mindset by practicing gratitude and reframing negative thoughts. Focus on growth and opportunity, even in adversity.
4. **Seek Inspiration**: Draw strength from resilient women who have faced and overcome significant challenges. Their stories can offer valuable guidance and motivation for your journey.
5. **Set Realistic Goals**: Break down big challenges into smaller, achievable steps. Setting manageable milestones can make the path forward feel less daunting.
6. **Embrace Change**: Resilience is linked to adaptability. Be flexible when circumstances shift and recognize that change often brings new opportunities.
7. **Healthy Lifestyle**: Prioritize your physical well-being. Proper nutrition, exercise, and sleep strengthen not just your body but your emotional resilience as well.
8. **Self-Care**: Engage in activities that replenish your energy, such as reading, being in nature, or pursuing a creative hobby. Self-care is essential to building resilience.

9. **Build a Support System**: Surround yourself with a network of people who provide encouragement and guidance during tough times.
10. **Learn from Setbacks**: Each setback offers a lesson. Instead of dwelling on past failures, use them as steppingstones to future success.
11. **Celebrate Small Wins**: Recognize and celebrate every achievement, no matter how small. Each victory strengthens your resilience and builds confidence.
12. **Practice Self-Compassion**: Treat yourself with kindness, especially in moments of self-doubt. Self-compassion is a cornerstone of resilience, helping you navigate challenges with grace.

Resilience is a journey of self-discovery and strength. It is about reaching within and using available resources to overcome adversity. As you cultivate resilience, you'll find that what once seemed insurmountable becomes an opportunity for growth and transformation.

The Transformative Power of Resilience

Resilience is not just about survival; it is a catalyst for personal growth and transformation. It allows us to approach life with renewed strength, confidence, and fearlessness. Here's how resilience can transform you:

1. **Confidence and Empowerment**: As you nurture resilience, you become more confident in your ability to face adversity, turning challenges into steppingstones for growth.
2. **Fearlessness**: Resilience fosters fearlessness. The ability to confront setbacks with courage becomes an integral part of your character.
3. **Adaptability**: Resilient individuals are adaptable, better equipped to navigate life's unpredictable changes, and more open to new opportunities.

4. **Mental Toughness**: Resilience builds mental toughness, allowing you to remain calm, composed, and clear-headed in difficult situations.
5. **Overcoming Fear of Failure**: Resilience helps you view failure as a learning experience rather than an endpoint. You become more willing to take risks and learn from them.
6. **Enhanced Critical Thinking**: Resilient individuals are effective problem solvers, viewing challenges as opportunities for creative solutions.
7. **Deeper Self-Understanding**: Resilience allows you to discover hidden strengths, confront weaknesses, and build a more profound connection with yourself.
8. **Fulfillment and Satisfaction**: Resilient people experience a deeper sense of fulfillment, appreciating their accomplishments and valuing the journey.
9. **Compassion**: Resilience nurtures compassion—for yourself and others—allowing you to offer support and encouragement to those facing challenges.
10. **Positive Influence**: As you transform through resilience, you become a source of inspiration for those around you, motivating them to face their own challenges with courage and resilience.

Resilience isn't just a defense mechanism; it's the key to unlocking personal growth, empowerment, and fearlessness. It reminds us that even in the face of adversity, we have the power to shape our destinies and become the strong, resilient women we aspire to be.

Inspiring Resilience in Others

Your journey of resilience has the power to inspire and empower those around you. Here are ways you can lead others on their paths to resilience:

1. **Lead by Example**: Demonstrating resilience through your own actions is the most powerful way to inspire others. Show them what strength looks like in the face of adversity.
2. **Storytelling**: Sharing your story can offer hope and guidance to others. By speaking openly about your challenges, you help others see that they too can overcome their obstacles.
3. **Mentoring**: Become a mentor to someone on their resilience journey. Your wisdom and insights can guide them through their challenges.
4. **Creating Safe Spaces**: Foster environments where people can explore their vulnerabilities and build resilience without fear of judgment.
5. **Promoting Inclusivity**: Resilience is for everyone. Recognize and celebrate the unique paths each person takes on their resilience journey.
6. **Supporting Causes**: By contributing to organizations that focus on empowerment and resilience, you help strengthen the collective journey of countless individuals.
7. **Lending a Helping Hand**: Offering support during someone else's challenging time can be a powerful testament to the strength of community and compassion.
8. **Amplifying Voices**: Share the stories of others who have demonstrated resilience, helping to highlight their strength and inspire a broader audience.
9. **Fostering Empathy**: Promote empathy for yourself and others, creating a compassionate environment that nurtures resilience.
10. **Advocating for Change**: Support changes in societal attitudes and systems that hinder resilience. Advocate for communities that are more inclusive, empathetic, and supportive.

By nurturing your resilience and sharing your journey, you become a beacon of hope and strength for others. Together, we can build a resilient community where each member is empowered to face adversity with courage and determination. **And in doing so, we create a world where resilience, strength, and empathy become the pillars of a more compassionate and empowered society.**

Interactive Questions for "Cultivating Resilience"

1. Self-Reflection and Understanding

- **Personal Inventory:** What are some personal strengths and weaknesses you've discovered about yourself through challenging experiences? How can these insights help you build resilience?
- **Trigger Points:** What specific situations or events tend to challenge your resilience the most? How do you typically respond, and what might you do differently in the future?

2. Embracing Change

- **Change Acceptance:** Think of a recent change in your life. How did you react initially? What steps did you take to adapt to this change, and what did you learn from the experience?
- **Future Readiness:** How can you better prepare yourself for future changes? What strategies can you implement to become more adaptable?

3. Developing Mental Toughness

- **Mental Resilience:** When faced with adversity, what techniques do you currently use to stay focused and positive? How effective are these techniques, and what could you improve?

- **Resilience Training:** What mental exercises or practices could you incorporate into your daily routine to enhance your mental toughness?

4. Seeking and Offering Support

- **Support Networks:** Who are the key people in your support network? How do they help you build resilience, and how can you reciprocate their support?
- **Support Strategies:** In what ways can you be more proactive in seeking help when needed? What are some new ways you might offer support to others facing challenges?

5. Embracing Failure and Learning from Setbacks

- **Failure as Feedback:** Reflect on a recent failure. What lessons did you learn from it? How can these lessons be applied to future challenges?
- **Growth Mindset:** How can you shift your perspective on failure to see it as an opportunity for growth rather than an endpoint?

6. Building Adaptability

- **Adaptability Assessment:** How do you handle unexpected changes or disruptions in your plans? What strategies have worked well for you in the past, and what new approaches could you try?
- **Flexibility Challenge:** Identify an area in your life where you struggle with adaptability. What specific steps can you take to become more flexible and open-minded?

7. Cultivating a Positive Mindset

- **Gratitude Practice:** What are three things you are grateful for today? How does focusing on gratitude impact your resilience?
- **Reframing Negative Thoughts:** Identify a recent negative thought or belief. How can you reframe it more positively and constructively?

8. Seeking Inspiration

- **Inspirational Stories:** Who are some resilient individuals you admire? What specific qualities or actions of theirs inspire you?
- **Learning from Others:** What lessons have you learned from the stories of resilient women featured in this chapter? How can you apply these lessons to your own life?

9. Setting Realistic Goals

- **Goal Breakdown:** Take a significant goal you have and break it down into smaller, manageable steps. What are these steps, and how will they help you achieve your larger goal?
- **Milestone Celebration:** How will you recognize and celebrate your progress toward this goal? Why is it important to acknowledge small wins along the way?

10. Practicing Self-Care

- **Self-Care Activities:** What activities or practices help you recharge and maintain your resilience? How often do you engage in these self-care activities?
- **Self-Care Plan:** Create a self-care plan for the next month. What specific actions will you take to ensure you are nurturing your well-being?

11. Celebrating Small Wins

- **Achievement Reflection:** What is a recent small win you've achieved? How did it contribute to your overall sense of accomplishment and confidence?
- **Victory Journal:** Start a journal to track and celebrate your small victories. How does reflecting on these successes impact your resilience?

12. Practicing Self-Compassion

- **Self-Compassion Exercise:** Reflect on a recent moment when you were hard on yourself. How can you practice self-compassion in a similar situation in the future?
- **Compassionate Dialogue:** How can you improve your inner dialogue to be more supportive and understanding during tough times?

13. Inspiring Resilience in Others

- **Leading by Example:** How can you model resilience for others in your life? What specific actions or attitudes would demonstrate this?
- **Mentorship Opportunities:** Are there opportunities for you to mentor or guide someone through their resilience journey? How can you offer support effectively?

14. Creating Safe Spaces

- **Supportive Environments:** How can you create safe spaces for others to explore their resilience? What characteristics or actions define a safe and supportive environment?
- **Empathy and Understanding:** How can fostering empathy and understanding contribute to creating a more resilient community?

Embracing the Journey of Resilience

We find ourselves standing at the intersection of reflection and action. Resilience is not merely a trait but a dynamic skill that each of us can develop and refine through our experiences and choices. It is the inner strength that allows us to rise above adversity, adapt to change, and emerge more powerful and self-aware.

We have explored the essential components of resilience, from accepting change and developing mental toughness to embracing failure and seeking support. Each lesson serves as a building block in the foundation of a resilient mindset, guiding us through life's inevitable challenges with grace and strength.

Key Takeaways:

1. **Acceptance of Change:** Embrace change as an inherent part of life, adapting with flexibility and an open mind.
2. **Mental Toughness:** Train your mind to remain strong, focused, and solution-oriented, avoiding overwhelm in the face of adversity.
3. **Seeking Support:** Recognize the strength in seeking help from others and build a robust support system to uplift and guide you.
4. **Embracing Failure:** View failure as a steppingstone to success, understanding that each setback is a lesson and an opportunity for growth.
5. **Learning from Setbacks:** Use challenges as chances to learn and evolve, examining the lessons within each difficulty.
6. **Staying Adaptable:** Foster adaptability by being open to change and flexible in your approach to life's twists and turns.

7. **Building a Support System:** Surround yourself with people who inspire and encourage you, reinforcing your resilience through a strong network.
8. **Positive Self-Talk:** Maintain a positive and self-compassionate inner dialogue, especially during moments of adversity.

As you continue on your journey of self-discovery, remember that resilience is not a destination but a continual practice. It is an ongoing process of building strength, embracing growth, and nurturing the inner power that lies within each of us.

Take the insights from this chapter and apply them to your daily life. Engage in self-reflection, seek inspiration, set realistic goals, and practice self-care. Celebrate your small victories and approach setbacks with a learning mindset. Each step you take towards cultivating resilience is a step towards a more empowered and fulfilling life.

Your journey is unique, and every challenge you face is an opportunity to uncover new strengths and perspectives. As you move forward, keep the lessons of resilience close to your heart and remain steadfast in your commitment to growth. Embrace the transformative power of resilience, and let it guide you toward a future filled with confidence, adaptability, and unwavering strength.

The path ahead may be filled with twists and turns, but with resilience as your companion, you have the power to navigate it with courage and grace. Continue to explore, reflect, and grow, and let your resilience shine brightly as a beacon of hope and strength. Your journey of self-discovery is just beginning, and the possibilities for growth and empowerment are limitless.

4-SETTING BOLD GOALS

Unleashing Your Inner Visionary

Setting goals is more than just creating a checklist for success; it's about embracing your limitless potential and daring to dream bigger than ever before. For unstoppable women, bold goals are more than mere targets — they're transformational journeys that allow them to live fully, with passion and purpose. In this chapter, we will dive into how to set bold, audacious goals that challenge you to grow, fuel your inner fire, and bring you closer to the extraordinary life you're meant to live.

Understanding Bold Goals

Bold goals are ambitious, sometimes daunting, and always inspiring. They differ from smaller, incremental goals because they stretch the boundaries of what you believe is possible. They require courage, a leap of faith, and a refusal to settle for mediocrity. Bold goals aren't just for achieving external success — they are about discovering your inner power, uncovering hidden strengths, and realizing the magnitude of your potential.

Why Bold Goals Matter

1. **Ignition of Passion:** Bold goals awaken something deep within you. When you set a goal that truly excites you, one that aligns with your core desires and values, it fuels a relentless passion that will drive you forward, even when the road gets tough.
2. **Clarity of Purpose:** The pursuit of bold goals brings focus. You aren't just drifting through life — you have a

clear, ambitious target. Bold goals force you to dig deep, to ask yourself what really matters and what you truly want to accomplish.

3. **Growth and Transformation:** The very nature of bold goals means they push you to become more than who you currently are. Along the way, you'll build resilience, sharpen your skills, and evolve in ways you never thought possible. It's in the pursuit of the bold that true transformation occurs.

Crafting Your Bold Goals

When setting bold goals, think big, think brave, and be unapologetic about your aspirations. Here's how to get started:

1. **Dream Limitlessly:** Bold goals begin with daring to dream without boundaries. What would you set out to achieve if you knew you couldn't fail? Let your imagination run wild and write down your most ambitious dreams — those that scare you and excite you all at once.
2. **Visualize Success:** Close your eyes and envision your life once you've achieved your bold goal. What does it look like? How do you feel? What impact have you made? This visualization not only helps solidify the goal in your mind but also makes it feel real and attainable.
3. **Define Your Why:** Bold goals require deep commitment, so it's essential to understand why the goal matters to you. Ask yourself: Why does this goal excite me? How does it align with my core values? What difference will it make in my life and the lives of others?
4. **Break It Down:** A bold goal can feel overwhelming at first. Break it down into smaller, actionable steps. Each

milestone achieved along the way will build your confidence and create a sense of momentum.

5. **Embrace the Uncertainty:** Bold goals come with uncertainty and risk. They will take you out of your comfort zone, and that's exactly where you need to be. Learn to embrace the discomfort, knowing it's part of the process. This journey is about stepping into the unknown with confidence.

Overcoming Fear and Doubt

With bold goals often come fear, doubt, and the voice in your head that says, *Who do you think you are to attempt this?* These feelings are normal and part of the journey, but they don't have to hold you back. Here's how to manage them:

1. **Turn Fear into Fuel:** Instead of letting fear paralyze you, let it fuel you. Fear is an indicator that you are pushing boundaries and stepping into new territory. Reframe it as a sign that you are moving in the right direction.

2. **Surround Yourself with Support:** You don't have to go after bold goals alone. Surround yourself with a tribe of like-minded women who believe in you, who will cheer you on, and who won't let you quit when the going gets tough.

3. **Celebrate Every Win:** Even small victories matter when pursuing bold goals. Every step forward deserves recognition. These small celebrations will keep your motivation alive and remind you of how far you've come.

4. **Fail Forward:** Expect that you will encounter setbacks along the way. Don't fear failure—embrace it as a powerful teacher. Each misstep brings you one step closer to achieving your goal, so learn, adjust, and keep moving.

The Personal Journey of Sarah Johnson: A Real-World Example

Sarah Johnson, a single mother of two from Atlanta, always had a dream of becoming a physician. But life had other plans for her — by the time she was 28, she found herself working two jobs just to make ends meet. The idea of going back to school, especially for something as demanding as medicine, seemed far-fetched. After all, she had kids to raise, bills to pay, and no support system to rely on. For years, she pushed the dream aside, believing it was no longer within her reach.

But one evening, after a particularly long shift at the diner where she worked, Sarah had a revelation. She realized that while she had been surviving, she wasn't truly living. The fire inside her had dimmed, and she longed to reignite it. Her dream of becoming a doctor still flickered in her heart. That night, she decided — she would chase her bold goal, no matter how impossible it seemed.

Step 1: Defining the Bold Goal

Sarah's bold goal was to become a doctor before her 40th birthday. It seemed impossible to many around her, but for Sarah, it became a beacon of hope and purpose. Her first step? Researching medical schools, even though she had no idea how she would afford the tuition or balance her responsibilities.

Step 2: Creating a Plan and Breaking It Down

Realizing that the journey would take years, Sarah broke the goal down into manageable chunks. First, she enrolled in a community college to take the necessary pre-med courses. She studied late at night after putting her kids to bed, determined to balance school, work, and motherhood.

Next, she set short-term milestones: completing her associate degree, applying for scholarships, and gaining experience by volunteering at a local clinic.

Step 3: Overcoming Challenges

There were countless obstacles. Financial strain, fatigue, and the emotional weight of juggling so much on her own led Sarah to moments of doubt. But her passion and the vision she had for her future kept her moving forward.

She surrounded herself with people who believed in her. Her kids became her biggest cheerleaders, and she connected with mentors at the clinic who guided her through the complex medical school application process.

Step 4: Reaching the Bold Goal

At age 37, after years of hard work, sacrifice, and sheer determination, Sarah was accepted into a medical program. She cried tears of joy, knowing that she was on the verge of transforming her life—not just for herself, but for her children, who had witnessed her tenacity.

Sarah graduated at 41, defying the odds and proving that bold goals are achievable no matter the challenges. Today, Dr. Sarah Johnson is a family physician, serving her community with pride. Her journey was long and arduous, but every step was worth it. She's a living example that bold goals, no matter how impossible they seem, can be achieved with courage, persistence, and an unwavering belief in oneself.

Staying Committed

Commitment to bold goals means showing up every day, even when it feels difficult. Here's how you can stay dedicated to your vision:

1. **Create Consistent Habits:** Integrate daily or weekly habits that support your goal. Whether it's dedicating time to learning a new skill, practicing mindfulness, or networking, consistency is key to keeping you on track.
2. **Reflect and Adjust:** Periodically take time to reflect on your progress. Are you getting closer to your goal? What challenges have you faced, and how can you overcome them moving forward? Make adjustments when needed but never lose sight of the bigger picture.
3. **Resilience is Everything:** Bold goals demand resilience. There will be setbacks, failures, and moments of self-doubt. But remember, resilience is not about never falling — it's about getting back up, time and again, with even greater resolve.

What is one small, consistent habit you can build that will support your bold goal? Start incorporating it into your daily routine.

As an unstoppable woman, the only limits you have are the ones you place on yourself. What bold goals will you set today that push the boundaries of what you once thought was possible?

Embrace the Journey of Boldness

Setting bold goals is an act of courage, a commitment to living a life of passion, purpose, and growth. Throughout this chapter, we've explored the transformative power of bold goals — how they ignite our inner fire, clarify our purpose, and push us to grow beyond our current limits. Bold goals aren't just about reaching a destination; they are about evolving into the strongest, most resilient version of yourself.

The journey won't always be easy. There will be moments of fear, doubt, and challenge. But every bold goal is worth the struggle because it forces you to tap into a well of inner strength you never knew you had. Remember that the setbacks you face along the way are not failures — they are lessons that will guide you toward success.

Key takeaways from this chapter:

- **Dream without limits:** Your bold goals should be rooted in your deepest desires. Don't hold back. The bigger the dream, the more powerful the transformation.
- **Visualize and define your why:** When you connect your goals to your core values, you ignite a passion that keeps you motivated through any obstacle.
- **Break it down:** Bold goals can seem overwhelming, but taking small, manageable steps ensures you're always moving forward.
- **Embrace uncertainty:** Growth only happens when you step out of your comfort zone and into the unknown.
- **Stay resilient and celebrate wins:** Every step counts. Celebrate your progress, and when setbacks occur, get back up stronger.

As you move forward, let this chapter serve as a reminder that you are capable of achieving more than you can imagine. Your bold goals are within reach, no matter how impossible they may seem today. Keep your vision clear, your steps consistent, and your spirit unshakable. You are an unstoppable woman with the power to shape your destiny.

Remember: the real reward is not just in achieving the goal, but in the woman, you become along the way.

Action Step: Take a moment to reflect on your bold goal. Write down one action you will take today to move closer to your vision, no matter how small. This is your journey, and every step forward matters.

Keep believing in yourself, keep setting bold goals, and never stop embracing your fire. Your journey of self-discovery and growth has only just begun. The world is waiting for your brilliance—keep moving forward.

Remember, as an unstoppable woman, the only limits you have are the ones you place on yourself. Setting bold goals is your way of breaking free from limitations and stepping into the greatness that awaits you. Embrace the fire within, and let it fuel your journey toward the extraordinary life you were born to create.

5. TAMING YOUR INNER CRITIC

Taming Your Inner Critic: Embracing Your True Potential

Every woman has an inner voice—a persistent narrator who scrutinizes every action, thought, and decision. For many, this voice manifests as a harsh critic, eroding confidence and fostering self-doubt. Taming this inner critic is crucial for embracing your true potential and stepping fully into your power. This chapter explores how to transform that critical voice into a supportive ally on your journey to becoming unstoppable.

Understanding the Inner Critic

The inner critic often stems from societal expectations, cultural conditioning, and personal experiences. From an early age, women receive messages about who they should be, how they should act, and what they should look like. These messages shape our subconscious and influence our inner dialogue.

The inner critic thrives on fear and insecurity, telling you that you're not good enough, smart enough, or strong enough. It whispers that you'll never succeed, that others are better, and that your dreams are unrealistic. Unchecked, this voice becomes a powerful barrier to your personal and professional growth.

Identifying the Inner Critic

The first step in taming your inner critic is recognizing when it speaks. Pay attention to the thoughts that arise when you face a challenge, seize an opportunity or experience vulnerability. Does your inner voice encourage you, or does it attempt to hold you back?

Common phrases from the inner critic might include:

- **"You're not ready for this."**
- **"What if you fail?"**
- **"They'll see right through you."**
- **"Who do you think you are?"**

These thoughts can feel automatic and ingrained, but they are learned responses and can be unlearned.

Challenging the Inner Critic

Once you've identified the voice of your inner critic, challenge it. Ask yourself:

- **Is this thought true?**
- **What evidence supports or contradicts this thought?**
- **Would I say this to a friend or loved one?**
- **What would I say to encourage someone else in this situation?**

Often, you'll find that the criticisms are unfounded or exaggerated. By questioning these thoughts, you begin to weaken the inner critic's hold on you.

Replacing Criticism with Compassion

To tame your inner critic, replace criticism with compassion. Speak to yourself as you would to a dear friend — someone you care about deeply and want to see thrive. Practice self-compassion by acknowledging your efforts, celebrating your successes, and being gentle with yourself when you stumble.

This shift requires consistent practice and a conscious effort to reframe negative thoughts into positive, supportive ones. When your inner critic says, **"You can't do this,"** respond with, **"I'm learning and growing, and I'm capable of great things."**

Building a Supportive Inner Dialogue

Creating a supportive inner dialogue involves more than silencing the critic; it's about nurturing an inner voice that uplifts and motivates you. Here are some strategies to build a more empowering internal conversation:

1. **Affirmations**: Start your day with positive affirmations that reflect your strengths and aspirations. Statements like "I am capable," "I am deserving of success," and "I embrace challenges as opportunities" can set a powerful tone for your day.
2. **Visualization**: Visualize yourself succeeding, overcoming obstacles, and achieving your goals. See yourself as the unstoppable force you are. This mental imagery helps counteract the negative images your inner critic might conjure.
3. **Gratitude**: Cultivate a habit of gratitude for your abilities, achievements, and growth. Focusing on what you're grateful for leaves less room for self-criticism.
4. **Mindfulness**: Practice mindfulness to stay present and grounded. Being fully engaged in the moment reduces the inner critic's influence.
5. **Self-Care**: Prioritize self-care as an essential part of taming your inner critic. Nurturing your body, mind, and spirit builds resilience against negative self-talk.

Surrounding Yourself with Positive Influences

The company you keep can significantly impact the strength of your inner critic. Surround yourself with people who uplift and inspire you, who believe in your potential, and who encourage you to pursue your dreams. Positive influences help drown out the critical voice and reinforce your belief in yourself.

Conversely, be mindful of relationships that fuel your inner critic. If certain people consistently doubt or belittle you, it may be time to reassess those connections. Protecting your energy and mental well-being is crucial as you work to tame your inner critic.

Embracing Imperfection

Perfectionism is a favorite weapon of the inner critic. It insists that anything less than perfect is a failure and that mistakes are unacceptable. This mindset can paralyze you, preventing you from taking steps that lead to growth and fulfillment.

Counter this by embracing imperfection as a natural part of life. Understand that mistakes are opportunities for learning and that progress is more important than perfection. Celebrate your efforts, regardless of the outcome, and recognize that every step forward is a victory.

Transforming the Critic into a Coach

Ultimately, the goal is not to silence your inner voice entirely but to transform it into a constructive, supportive force. Think of it as turning your inner critic into an inner coach—one that provides constructive feedback rather than destructive criticism.

An inner coach acknowledges areas for improvement with kindness and encouragement. It says, "You did well, and here's how you can do even better next time," instead of, "You messed up again."

Taming Your Inner Critic: Embracing Your True Potential

Every woman has an inner voice—a persistent narrator who scrutinizes every action, thought, and decision. For many, this voice manifests as a harsh critic, eroding confidence and fostering self-doubt. Taming this inner critic is crucial for embracing your true potential and stepping fully into your power. This chapter explores how to transform that critical voice into a supportive ally on your journey to becoming unstoppable.

Understanding the Inner Critic

The inner critic often originates from a blend of societal expectations, cultural conditioning, and personal experiences. From an early age, women are inundated with messages about who they should be, how they should act, and what they should look like. These messages infiltrate our subconscious and shape our inner dialogue.

The inner critic thrives on fear and insecurity. It tells you that you're not good enough, smart enough, or strong enough. It whispers that you'll never succeed, that others are better, and that your dreams are unrealistic. If left unchecked, this voice becomes a formidable barrier to your personal and professional growth.

Identifying the Inner Critic

The first step in taming your inner critic is recognizing when it speaks. Pay close attention to your thoughts when faced with challenges, new opportunities, or moments of vulnerability. Is your inner voice encouraging you, or is it attempting to hold you back?

Common phrases from the inner critic might include:

- **"You're not ready for this."**
- **"What if you fail?"**
- **"They'll see right through you."**
- **"Who do you think you are?"**

These thoughts may feel automatic and ingrained, but they are learned responses and can be unlearned.

Challenging the Inner Critic

Once you've identified the voice of your inner critic, it's time to challenge it. Ask yourself:

- **Is this thought true?** Examine whether there is factual evidence to support or refute the criticism.
- **What evidence supports or contradicts this** negative **thought?** Look for concrete examples that challenge the belief.
- **Would I say this to a friend or loved one?** Consider whether the criticism is something you would direct toward someone you care about.
- **What would I say to encourage someone else in this situation?** Think about how you would support and motivate another person facing similar doubts.

Often, you'll find that these criticisms are unfounded or exaggerated. By questioning these thoughts, you can begin to weaken the inner critic's hold on you.

Replacing Criticism with Compassion

To tame your inner critic, replace criticism with compassion. Speak to yourself as you would to a dear friend — someone you care about deeply and want to see thrive. Practice self-compassion by acknowledging your efforts, celebrating your successes, and being gentle with yourself when you stumble.

This shift requires consistent practice and a conscious effort to reframe negative thoughts into positive, supportive ones. When your inner critic says, "You can't do this," respond with, "I'm learning and growing, and I'm capable of great things."

Building a Supportive Inner Dialogue

Creating a supportive inner dialogue involves more than silencing the critic; it's about nurturing an inner voice that uplifts and motivates you. Here are strategies to build a more empowering internal conversation:

1. **Affirmations**: Start your day with positive affirmations that reflect your strengths and aspirations. Statements like "I am capable," "I am deserving of success," and "I embrace challenges as opportunities" set a powerful tone for your day.
2. **Visualization**: Visualize yourself succeeding, overcoming obstacles, and achieving your goals. See yourself as the unstoppable force you are. This mental imagery helps counteract the negative images your inner critic might conjure.
3. **Gratitude**: Cultivate a habit of gratitude for your abilities, achievements, and growth. Focusing on what you're grateful for leaves less room for self-criticism and fosters a more positive mindset.
4. **Mindfulness**: Practice mindfulness to stay present and grounded. Being fully engaged now reduces the inner critic's influence and helps you respond to challenges with clarity.
5. **Self-Care**: Prioritize self-care as an essential part of taming your inner critic. Nurturing your body, mind, and spirit builds resilience against negative self-talk. Regular self-care practices — such as exercise, hobbies, and relaxation techniques — are vital for maintaining mental and emotional well-being.

Surrounding Yourself with Positive Influences

The company you keep can significantly impact the strength of your inner critic. Surround yourself with people who uplift and inspire you, who believe in your potential, and who encourage you to pursue your dreams. Positive influences help drown out the critical voice and reinforce your belief in yourself.

Conversely, be mindful of relationships that fuel your inner critic. If certain people consistently doubt or belittle you, it may be time to reassess those connections. Protecting your energy and mental well-being is crucial as you work to tame your inner critic. Building a network of supportive individuals can create a nurturing environment where you feel empowered to thrive.

Embracing Imperfection

Perfectionism is a favorite weapon of the inner critic. It insists that anything less than perfect is a failure and that mistakes are unacceptable. This mindset can paralyze you, preventing you from taking steps that lead to growth and fulfillment.

Counter this by embracing imperfection as a natural part of life. Understand that mistakes are opportunities for learning and that progress is more important than perfection. Celebrate your efforts, regardless of the outcome, and recognize that every step forward is a victory. Accepting imperfection allows you to pursue your goals with greater courage and resilience.

Transforming the Critic into a Coach

Ultimately, the goal is not to silence your inner voice entirely but to transform it into a constructive, supportive force. Think of it as turning your inner critic into an inner coach—one that provides constructive feedback rather than destructive criticism.

An inner coach acknowledges areas for improvement with kindness and encouragement. It says, "You did well, and here's how you can do even better next time," instead of, "You messed up again." This approach fosters a growth mindset and encourages continuous improvement.

Reflection Questions:

1. **Recognizing Your Inner Critic:**
    - Can you recall a recent moment when your inner critic held you back? What did it say, and how did it affect your actions or decisions?
    - How often do you hear your inner critic when you try something new or take on a challenge? What triggers it the most in your life?
2. **Challenging Negative Thoughts:**
    - Think of a negative thought you've had about yourself recently. What evidence supports or contradicts this thought?
    - If a friend were in your situation, what would you tell her to encourage and support her? How can you apply that same advice to yourself?
3. **Rewriting Your Inner Dialogue:**
    - Write down three common phrases your inner critic uses. Now, rewrite them as positive affirmations that are both encouraging and realistic.
    - How do you typically react to setbacks or mistakes? What would your inner coach say instead to help you grow from the experience?
4. **Embracing Imperfection:**
    - In what areas of your life do you feel pressured to be perfect? How can you reframe these areas to focus on progress and learning instead of perfection?
    - Share a time when you made a mistake but learned something valuable from it. How can you apply this lesson moving forward?
5. **Nurturing Self-Compassion:**

- o How do you currently practice self-compassion? If it's not something you often do, what's one small way you can start being kinder to yourself?
- o What positive qualities or strengths do you often overlook in yourself? List three things you're proud of accomplishing recently.

6. **Surrounding Yourself with Positivity:**
   - o Who in your life makes you feel supported and empowered? How can you spend more time with these positive influences?
   - o Are there any relationships or environments that fuel your inner critic? What steps can you take to protect your energy and well-being?

7. **Visualization and Affirmations:**
   - o What's one challenge or goal you're working toward right now? Visualize yourself succeeding. How do you feel in that moment of success, and what steps can you take to get there?
   - o Create a personal affirmation that speaks to your strengths and goals. How can you incorporate it into your daily routine to help shift your inner dialogue?

8. **Transforming Criticism into Constructive Feedback:**
   - o Think of a recent time when your inner critic was particularly harsh. How could you reframe that criticism into constructive feedback that helps you grow?
   - o What specific qualities or skills would you like to develop further? How can your "inner coach" guide you in strengthening these areas?

Embracing Your Fire

Taming your inner critic is not an overnight transformation, but a continuous, empowering journey toward embracing your true self. It's about reclaiming your voice, recognizing your worth, and shifting from self-criticism to self-compassion. By identifying and challenging the negative thoughts that hold you back, you open the door to growth, confidence, and resilience. Every step you take toward silencing that inner critic is a step toward unlocking your full potential.

Remember, your journey to self-love and empowerment is uniquely yours, and every moment of progress is worth celebrating. You are capable of rewriting the narrative in your mind. The more you replace self-doubt with affirmations, self-compassion, and supportive inner dialogue, the more unstoppable you become.

Summary and Encouragement:

**In this chapter, we explored the powerful steps to taming your inner critic:**

- **Recognizing your inner critic** is the first step to understanding how self-doubt manifests in your thoughts.
- **Challenging negative self-talk** allows you to reframe limiting beliefs with self-empowerment and encouragement.
- **Embracing self-compassion** helps you replace harsh judgments with kindness and understanding toward yourself.
- **Rewriting your inner dialogue** gives you the ability to transform criticism into affirmations that uplift you.

- **Letting go of perfectionism** frees you from unrealistic expectations, encouraging progress and resilience over flawlessness.
- **Surrounding yourself with positivity** creates an environment that nurtures your self-worth and counters negative influences.
- **Building self-respect** reinforces your boundaries, celebrates your worth, and strengthens your confidence.

Know that each moment you invest in silencing your inner critic is a testament to your strength and self-love. By turning your inner critic into an ally, you unlock a life full of possibilities, driven by the belief that you are enough—and more than capable of achieving your dreams.

This journey will take patience, practice, and persistence, but every step forward is a victory. Keep nurturing your fire, embracing your unique qualities, and trusting that you are unstoppable. Your path to self-empowerment is unfolding, and the best is yet to come.

6. BUILDING UNSHAKEABLE CONFIDENCE

A Woman's Journey to Empowerment and Resilience

In a world that often challenges women's worth, abilities, and potential, developing unshakable confidence is more important than ever. Confidence is not a trait that comes naturally to everyone, nor is it an end state. It is a lifelong journey, one that every woman must embark on to unlock her fullest potential and lead a life rich in purpose, joy, and fulfillment.

This chapter delves deeply into the transformative power of unshakable confidence. It explores how this confidence—rooted not in external validation, but in self-worth and inner resilience—empowers women to navigate the complexities of life with grace, poise, and unrelenting strength. More than a simple self-help guide, this chapter is a call to action: to recognize your unique strengths, face your fears, embrace your individuality, and pursue your dreams fearlessly.

1. The True Essence of Unshakable Confidence

Unshakable confidence transcends superficial self-esteem. It is an unwavering belief in your abilities, resilience, and worth—regardless of the obstacles you face. This confidence is not determined by success or accolades, nor is it contingent on how others perceive you. Rather, it is rooted in the profound realization that you possess the capability, power, and perseverance to achieve anything you set your mind to.

Many women struggle to develop this kind of deep, inner confidence because society often imposes external standards of success and beauty. Women are judged by their appearance, accomplishments, and adherence to societal expectations. But unshakable confidence flourishes when a woman recognizes her intrinsic value — when she knows that her worth is not defined by how others see her, but by how she sees herself.

Confidence is not the absence of doubt or fear; it is the determination to move forward despite them. It is the ability to stand tall in the face of adversity, trusting in your inner resources to weather any storm. This type of confidence doesn't just open doors — it transforms how you walk through them, allowing you to face life's challenges with resilience, adaptability, and grace.

2. Embracing and Celebrating Your Strengths

One of the first steps in developing unshakable confidence is recognizing and owning your unique strengths. Too often, women downplay their abilities or shy away from acknowledging their achievements. This may stem from societal conditioning, which encourages modesty and discourages women from "bragging" about their accomplishments. However, understanding and embracing your strengths is a critical part of building confidence.

It's essential to take the time to reflect on your skills, talents, and accomplishments. What are the qualities that make you uniquely you? What challenges have you overcome, and how have those experiences shaped you into the person you are today? Writing down your achievements and acknowledging your progress can be an empowering exercise. This practice allows you to cultivate a deeper sense of self-awareness and appreciate your capabilities.

By recognizing your strengths, you lay the foundation for unshakable confidence. When you know what you bring to the table, you become less concerned with seeking validation from others. You begin to trust in your judgment and abilities, which empowers you to take on new challenges with confidence and determination.

3. The Power of Self-Appreciation

Self-appreciation is often misunderstood as vanity or self-centeredness, but it is an essential component of unshakable confidence. When you appreciate yourself—your talents, your achievements, and even your imperfections—you strengthen your sense of self-worth. This, in turn, fuels your confidence and allows you to navigate life with greater ease and self-assurance.

Appreciating yourself means acknowledging that you are enough, just as you are. It means letting go of the need for perfection and embracing the reality that you are a work in progress. Self-appreciation also involves treating yourself with kindness, patience, and compassion. Instead of criticizing yourself for mistakes or perceived shortcomings, practice self-compassion by recognizing that everyone makes mistakes—and that those mistakes are growth opportunities.

When you appreciate yourself, you are less likely to seek validation from others. You stop comparing yourself to others and start focusing on your journey. This shift in mindset is crucial for building unshakable confidence, as it allows you to trust in your abilities and decisions without relying on external approval.

4. Building Confidence from Within: The Importance of Self-Validation

In a world where external validation is often seen as the measure of success, it's easy to fall into the trap of seeking approval from others. However, true confidence comes from within—it is built on the foundation of self-validation. When you rely on others to validate your worth, you give away your power. But when you learn to validate yourself, you reclaim that power and strengthen your confidence.

Self-validation means trusting in your own judgment, acknowledging your own accomplishments, and recognizing your own value. It means being able to stand firm in your decisions and beliefs, even when others disagree. This kind of inner confidence is what allows you to stay grounded and focused, even in the face of criticism or rejection.

To cultivate self-validation, start by affirming your worth and abilities. Practice positive self-talk and remind yourself of your strengths and accomplishments. When you achieve something, take the time to celebrate it—don't wait for others to acknowledge your success. By consistently validating yourself, you build the kind of unshakable confidence that cannot be shaken by external circumstances.

5. Overcoming Self-Doubt: A Pathway to Confidence

Self-doubt is one of the biggest obstacles to confidence. It creeps in when you least expect it, making you question your abilities, your worth, and your decisions. However, overcoming self-doubt is possible, and it is a critical part of building unshakable confidence.

The first step in overcoming self-doubt is recognizing it for what it is: a mental habit that can be changed. Self-doubt often stems from fear—fear of failure, fear of rejection, or fear of the unknown. To combat self-doubt, challenge the negative thoughts that fuel it. Ask yourself: Is this doubt based on facts, or is it rooted in fear? Are these negative thoughts helping me, or are they holding me back?

Once you've identified the sources of your self-doubt, work to replace them with more positive, empowering beliefs. Focus on your past successes and the challenges you've already overcome. Remind yourself of your strengths and capabilities.

Over time, this practice of positive self-talk will diminish the power of self-doubt and help you develop the confidence needed to face any challenge.

6. The Importance of Setting and Achieving Goals

Setting and achieving goals is one of the most effective ways to build confidence. Each time you accomplish a goal—whether big or small—you reinforce your belief in your abilities. This, in turn, strengthens your confidence and motivates you to pursue even greater challenges.

When setting goals, it's important to start small. Break down larger goals into smaller, more manageable steps. This not only makes the goal seem less daunting, but it also allows you to experience the satisfaction of achieving smaller milestones along the way. Each small win builds momentum and reinforces your confidence in your ability to succeed.

It's also important to celebrate your achievements, no matter how small they may seem. Recognize that each step forward is a victory and take the time to acknowledge your progress. Celebrating your successes reinforces your belief in your capabilities and sets a powerful precedent for future accomplishments.

7. Assertiveness: A Key Component of Confidence

Assertiveness is a vital skill for building unshakable confidence. It involves standing up for yourself, communicating your needs and boundaries clearly, and expressing your thoughts and opinions with confidence. Assertiveness is not about being aggressive or domineering— it's about being clear, direct, and respectful in your communication.

Many women struggle with assertiveness because they fear being perceived as "bossy" or "difficult." However, learning to be assertive is essential for building confidence and maintaining healthy relationships. Assertiveness allows you to advocate for yourself, set boundaries, and ensure that your needs are met—all of which are crucial for maintaining your confidence and self-worth.

To practice assertiveness, start by being clear about what you want or need in any given situation. Use "I" statements to express your feelings and needs and be direct without being confrontational. Over time, as you become more comfortable asserting yourself, you'll find that your confidence grows as well.

8. Body Positivity and Confidence

Confidence is not just a mental state—it's also about how you feel in your own body. Body positivity is a critical component of unshakable confidence, as it involves embracing your body for what it is: **strong, resilient, and beautiful in its unique way.**

Too often, women are taught to view their bodies through the lens of societal standards of beauty, which can lead to feelings of inadequacy and insecurity. However, true confidence comes from shifting the focus away from how your body looks and toward what it can do.

Building Unshakable Confidence: A Journey of Empowerment

Embarking on the journey to unshakable confidence is one of the most empowering paths a woman can take. It's not about arrogance or vanity, but about deeply understanding your value, embracing your unique strengths, and developing the inner resilience to face any challenge life throws at you. In this chapter, we explore the vital importance of unshakable confidence and how it transforms the way you navigate the world—with poise, grace, and power.

1. Defining Unshakable Confidence

Unshakable confidence is more than just a fleeting sense of self-esteem. It's the deep, unwavering belief in your abilities, self-worth, and the undeniable value you bring to the world. This confidence allows you to stand strong in the face of adversity, trust your instincts, and lead a life driven by your true purpose. It's not contingent on success or others' opinions; rather, it's an inner assurance that you can weather any storm.

2. Recognize and Own Your Strengths

To cultivate unshakable confidence, you must first acknowledge and celebrate your strengths, talents, and the qualities that set you apart. Too often, we downplay our achievements or compare ourselves to others. But confidence thrives when you embrace the reality that you are capable, worthy, and deserving of success. Write down your accomplishments and reflect on the challenges you've already overcome—this will reinforce your sense of capability and fuel your confidence moving forward.

3. Embrace Self-Appreciation

Appreciating yourself is not selfish—it's essential. Unshakable confidence grows when you fully accept and love yourself, including your imperfections. Understand that no one is perfect, and your quirks, mistakes, and missteps are part of what makes you uniquely you. Cultivate self-compassion by treating yourself as you would a close friend, with kindness, patience, and grace.

4. Self-Validation: Build from Within

Stop relying on external validation to determine your worth. Unshakable confidence comes from self-validation, the recognition that your value isn't defined by others' approval but by your own beliefs about yourself. Practice affirming your accomplishments, decisions, and boundaries. Trust yourself to be enough without the need for constant reinforcement from others.

5. Overcome Self-Doubt

Self-doubt is the enemy of confidence, but it can be defeated. When doubt creeps in, challenge it. Ask yourself: Is this doubt based on facts, or is it rooted in fear? Replace negative thoughts with affirmations of your abilities and past successes. Building this habit of positive self-talk will diminish the power of self-doubt over time and fortify your confidence.

6. Set and Achieve Goals: Small Wins Matter

Confidence thrives on accomplishment, and every small win builds momentum. Setting achievable goals—both large and small—fuels your self-belief. Each time you complete a task or hit a milestone, no matter how minor, you're reinforcing the idea that you are capable of achieving success. Celebrate these victories, and they will serve as steppingstones to larger accomplishments.

7. Practice Assertiveness: Speak Your Truth

Assertiveness is a vital skill for building confidence. It's the ability to communicate your needs, desires, and boundaries clearly and respectfully without fear or hesitation. Learning to express yourself assertively, whether in personal relationships or professional settings, reinforces the idea that your voice matters, and it deserves to be heard.

8. Embrace Body Positivity

Confidence is not just mental; it's physical as well. Unshakable confidence includes feeling comfortable in your skin and embracing your body for its strength, resilience, and beauty. Shift the focus from how your body looks to what it can do. Celebrate your body's ability to move, heal, and carry you through life's challenges.

9. Visualize Success: See It Before You Achieve It

Visualization is a powerful tool for building unshakable confidence. By imagining yourself succeeding—whether in your career, relationships, or personal goals—you're training your brain to believe that success is possible. Picture yourself overcoming obstacles and achieving your dreams. This mental rehearsal builds your belief in your capabilities and prepares you to face real-world challenges with greater assurance.

10. Embrace Failure as a Path to Growth

Failure is not the opposite of success—it's a steppingstone to it. Unshakable confidence is built when you shift your mindset around failure, viewing it as an opportunity for growth and learning rather than a reflection of your worth. Each setback offers valuable lessons and brings you one step closer to achieving your goals. When you can embrace failure as part of the process, your confidence will remain unshaken by the inevitable bumps in the road.

11. Prioritize Mental and Emotional Health

Your mental and emotional well-being are the foundations of unshakable confidence. Confidence thrives in a mind that is calm, clear, and resilient. Make self-care a priority, whether through mindfulness, meditation, journaling, or therapy. Taking care of your emotional health allows you to show up in the world with confidence and maintain that confidence even in stressful situations.

12. Surround Yourself with Support

Confidence doesn't develop in isolation. Surround yourself with people who believe in you, encourage you, and uplift your spirit. Seek out mentors, friends, and a community that sees your potential and pushes you toward your goals. Having a support system reinforces your belief in yourself, providing a safe space to grow and flourish.

13. Act: Confidence Is Built in Motion

Unshakable confidence is not just about how you feel; it's about what you do. Acting, especially in the face of fear, is one of the most effective ways to build and reinforce confidence. Start with small steps outside of your comfort zone, and as you achieve each one, you'll gain the courage to tackle bigger challenges. Remember, confidence is not the absence of fear—it's the willingness to move forward despite it.

14. Celebrate Your Successes—Big and Small

Women often downplay their achievements, but it's crucial to recognize and celebrate your wins. Acknowledging your success reinforces your belief in your abilities and sets a powerful precedent for future accomplishments. Take the time to celebrate both your big milestones and smaller victories, as each one contributes to your overall sense of confidence.

15. Continuous Learning and Growth

Confidence grows when you commit to learning and evolving. Never stop seeking knowledge and opportunities to expand your skills. Whether it's through formal education, personal development, or life experiences, continuous learning helps you stay adaptable, resilient, and confident in your ability to handle whatever comes your way.

1. Understanding Confidence

- How do you personally define confidence? Do you see it as a fixed trait or something that can be developed over time?
- Can you recall a time when you felt truly confident? What factors contributed to that feeling?

2. Recognizing Strengths

- What are three strengths or abilities you possess that you are most proud of? How have these strengths helped you in challenging situations?
- Why do you think many women tend to downplay their achievements? Have you experienced this, and how did it affect your self-confidence?

3. Self-Appreciation

- In what ways do you currently practice self-appreciation? If you don't, what are some ways you could begin?
- What does self-appreciation mean to you? How is it different from being self-critical?

4. Building Confidence from Within

- How often do you seek validation from others? How do you feel when you don't receive the validation you expect?
- Think of a recent accomplishment. Did you celebrate it, or wait for others to acknowledge it? How would celebrating yourself more often impact your self-esteem?

5. Overcoming Self-Doubt

- What are some recurring doubts you experience about yourself? How do you typically respond to these doubts?
- How do you differentiate between constructive self-criticism and unproductive self-doubt? What strategies could help you manage self-doubt more healthily?

6. Setting and Achieving Goals

- What is one personal or professional goal you are currently working toward? How does achieving this goal connect with building your confidence?
- Reflect on a recent goal you've accomplished. How did it feel to achieve it, and how did it impact your sense of self-worth?

7. Assertiveness and Boundaries

- In what situations do you find it most challenging to assert yourself? How does this affect your confidence in those moments?
- How would practicing assertiveness more regularly benefit your personal or professional life? What steps could you take to become more assertive?

8. Body Positivity and Confidence

- How do you currently feel about your body? In what ways do societal standards influence those feelings?
- What are some ways you can shift your focus from how your body looks to what it is capable of? How might this change impact on your overall confidence?

9. Reflection and Growth

- What is the most significant challenge you face in building unshakable confidence? How do you plan to overcome it?
- How can you begin to implement the concepts of self-appreciation, goal setting, or assertiveness into your daily life starting today?

Unshakable Confidence — Your Foundation for an Empowered Life

Unshakable confidence is not just a trait but a powerful force that propels you forward in life, enabling you to face challenges with courage, embrace your uniqueness, and trust in your inherent worth. It's about cultivating resilience, acknowledging your strengths, and stepping into your power with unwavering belief in yourself. This chapter has taken you through the essential pillars of unshakable confidence: from self-awareness and self-appreciation to goal setting, assertiveness, and overcoming self-doubt.

Each of these elements is a building block that contributes to your growth and personal empowerment. Confidence is not something you "arrive at" but a lifelong journey — a practice that deepens with every risk you take, every failure you learn from, and every success you own. As you embark on this path, remember that the goal isn't perfection. Instead, it's about embracing your journey, celebrating progress, and allowing yourself the grace to grow.

Unshakable confidence transforms not only how you perceive yourself but also how you engage with the world around you. As you continue developing this inner strength, you will find that your confidence has a ripple effect, influencing your relationships, career, and ability to inspire others. You will become a leader in your own life and a beacon for those around you.

Summary and Key Takeaways:

1. **Confidence is Cultivated:** True confidence comes from within and is built over time through self-awareness, self-appreciation, and a deep belief in your worth and capabilities.
2. **Embrace Your Strengths and Imperfections:** Recognizing and celebrating your strengths is vital, but so is accepting your imperfections. Confidence grows when you embrace both, allowing yourself to be human and imperfect.
3. **Self-Validation Over External Validation:** Learning to validate yourself and not rely on others for affirmation is key to building unshakable confidence. Your worth is inherent and not dependent on external opinions.
4. **Overcoming Self-Doubt:** Self-doubt is a natural part of life, but it doesn't have to define you. Challenge negative thoughts, replace them with affirmations, and trust in your ability to grow and succeed.
5. **Set and Achieve Goals:** Confidence is reinforced by setting goals, taking action, and celebrating every step of progress, no matter how small. Each goal achieved is a testament to your capabilities.
6. **Assertiveness and Boundaries:** Practicing assertiveness is crucial for building confidence. It allows you to communicate your needs and boundaries with respect for yourself and others.
7. **Body Positivity:** Confidence extends to how you feel about your body. By embracing body positivity, you strengthen your self-image and accept your body as a source of strength and resilience.
8. **Embrace Failure as Growth:** Failure is not an end but an opportunity to learn and grow. Embracing this

perspective will empower you to take risks and keep moving forward without fear.

9. **Resilience and Mental Health:** Confidence is rooted in resilience and mental well-being. Prioritize practices that nourish your mind and emotional health, such as mindfulness, therapy, or self-care routines.

Carry forward the knowledge that confidence is a practice — an ongoing journey of self-discovery, growth, and empowerment. Embrace each step, challenge, and success as a part of your evolution toward becoming the best version of yourself. Continue this journey of self-discovery with the understanding that every woman, including you, has the capacity for unshakable confidence. Believe in yourself, stand tall in your worth, and let your inner fire lead the way. You are unstoppable.

7. Effective Time Management

Mastering Time – The Fuel for Your Fire

In the journey toward becoming an unstoppable woman, mastering time is a crucial element. Time is the most precious resource we have—once it's gone, we can never reclaim it. Yet, for many of us, it feels as if time is constantly slipping through our fingers, leaving us feeling overwhelmed and behind. In a world of endless distractions, demands, and expectations, how can we take control of our time and use it as a force for transformation? The answer lies in learning how to master time, not just for efficiency, but for fueling your inner fire— your passion, purpose, and vision for a life well-lived.

Time management is not about squeezing more tasks into your day. It's about making intentional choices that align with your deepest values and long-term goals. By doing so, you transform your days from a series of chaotic events into a purposeful path toward the life you've always dreamed of. This chapter is dedicated to equipping you with the mindset, tools, and strategies to turn time into your greatest asset.

The Mindset Shift: Time as Your Ally, Not Your Enemy

One of the biggest barriers to mastering time is the way we perceive it. For many, time feels like an enemy—an obstacle to overcome. We feel rushed, anxious, and as though we never have enough of it. This mindset is not only stressful, but it also blinds us to the true potential that time offers. The first step toward mastery is shifting your perspective. Time is not your enemy; it's your ally.

Think of time as the raw material for creating the life you want. It's a neutral resource, and how you use it determines its value. When you adopt a mindset of abundance toward time, you stop worrying about how little of it you have and start focusing on how to make the most of it. This shift in mindset allows you to approach each day with clarity and purpose rather than panic and stress.

Reflection Question: How do you currently view time—as an enemy or an ally? How can you shift your perspective to see time as a powerful resource?

Conducting a Time Audit: Where is Your Time Going?

Before you can master time, you need to know where it's going. Most of us have a vague idea of how we spend our days, but without a clear picture, it's impossible to make meaningful changes. Conducting a time audit is a critical step in understanding your habits, identifying time leaks, and discovering opportunities for improvement.

Start by tracking every activity you engage in for a full week. This includes work tasks, personal activities, leisure time, and even mundane tasks like commuting, cooking, and cleaning. Break your day down into 15-minute or 30-minute intervals. While this may seem tedious, it's an eye-opening exercise that reveals where your time is being spent and where it's being wasted.

Once you have the data, analyze it. Are there certain activities that take up more time than you realized? Are there tasks you can delegate or eliminate? Is your time being spent in ways that align with your goals and values?

Reflection Question: What patterns do you notice in your time audit? Are there activities that no longer serve you and can be minimized?

Clarifying Your Priorities: The North Star of Time Management

Time mastery is rooted in clarity. Without a clear understanding of your priorities, it's easy to get lost in the whirlwind of daily demands. What truly matters to you? What are the key areas of your life that you want to nurture and grow? Defining your priorities provides a compass for your decisions, helping you allocate time to the things that matter most.

One effective way to clarify your priorities is by using the "Wheel of Life" exercise. Imagine a wheel divided into sections, each representing a different area of life: career, health, relationships, personal growth, finances, fun, and spirituality. Rate your satisfaction in each area on a scale of 1-10. This will give you a visual representation of where you're thriving and where you may need to invest more time and energy.

Once you've identified your key priorities, the next step is to align your daily actions with these areas. This is where many people struggle—knowing what's important is one thing, but consistently prioritizing those areas is another. To overcome this challenge, practice intentional time blocking, where you set aside specific chunks of time each day or week for activities that align with your top priorities.

Reflection Question: What are your top three priorities in life right now? How much time are you currently devoting to them?

The Power of Strategic Planning: Aligning Your Goals with Time

Effective time management requires both big-picture thinking and daily planning. Start by setting long-term goals that reflect your life's purpose and passions. Break those goals down into medium-term objectives (quarterly or monthly) and short-term tasks (weekly or daily). This layered approach ensures that your daily actions are consistently moving you toward your larger vision.

- **Yearly Planning:** Define your major goals and intentions for the year. What do you want to achieve in your career, personal life, and health? Create a clear vision for each area.
- **Quarterly Planning:** Every three months, review your yearly goals and create a specific action plan for the next 90 days. Break your big goals into smaller, manageable projects.
- **Monthly Planning:** At the start of each month, outline the tasks and milestones that will bring you closer to your quarterly goals. Set monthly themes or focus areas.
- **Weekly Planning:** Every Sunday, plan your week. Identify your top priorities, block out time for important tasks, and schedule any appointments or commitments.
- **Daily Planning:** Each morning or the night before, create a simple to-do list for the day. Include your top three non-negotiable tasks — these are the things that, if completed, will make the day a success.

By aligning your daily and weekly actions with your larger goals, you create a seamless connection between the present moment and your long-term vision. You ensure that every hour you spend is contributing to something meaningful.

Reflection Question: How can you break down your big goals into actionable, time-bound tasks that align with your daily schedule?

Overcoming Procrastination: From Hesitation to Action

Procrastination is one of the biggest obstacles to time mastery. We all experience it—those moments when we avoid starting a task, even though we know it's important. But procrastination is not a sign of laziness; it's often a signal of deeper fears, doubts, or overwhelm. To overcome procrastination, you must understand its root causes and develop strategies for pushing through hesitation.

- **Perfectionism:** If you're waiting for the "perfect time" to start something, remember that perfection is an illusion. Taking imperfect action is better than waiting for ideal conditions.
- **Fear of Failure:** If you're afraid of failing, remind yourself that failure is part of growth. Every setback is an opportunity to learn and improve.
- **Overwhelm:** If a task feels too big, break it down into smaller steps. Focus on the first small action you can take right now.

One of the most effective techniques for combating procrastination is the **"5-Minute Rule."** Commit to working on a task for just five minutes. Once you get started, you'll often find it easier to continue. Momentum builds from action, no matter how small.

Reflection Question: What tasks have you been procrastinating on? How can you break them down and take the first small step today?

Mastering the Art of Delegation: Letting Go to Grow

As women, we often take on the role of juggling multiple responsibilities, trying to do everything ourselves. However, one of the most powerful time management skills is delegation. Learning to delegate not only frees up your time, but it also allows you to focus on what truly matters and where your unique strengths lie.

Delegation doesn't mean passing off your responsibilities; it means empowering others to help you achieve your goals. Whether it's outsourcing tasks in your business, asking for help at home, or enlisting the support of colleagues or family members, delegation is essential for time mastery.

To delegate effectively, start by identifying the tasks that drain your energy or don't align with your strengths. Then, find the right people or resources to take on these tasks. Communicate, set expectations, and trust others to deliver. By letting go of control in certain areas, you create space for growth in the areas that fuel your fire.

Reflection Question: What tasks can you delegate or outsource to free up more time for your high-priority goals?

The Power of Rituals and Boundaries: Guarding Your Time Fiercely

In a world of constant demands, learning to guard your time fiercely is a critical skill. This involves setting boundaries with others and with yourself. When you don't protect your time, it gets eaten away by distractions, interruptions, and obligations that don't align with your goals.

One way to protect your time is by creating rituals that anchor your day. These are non-negotiable practices that help you stay grounded and focused. Whether it's a morning routine that sets the tone for your day, or a wind-down ritual that helps you transition from work to rest, rituals provide structure and intention.

Equally important is learning to say "no." saying no is not a rejection of others; it's a powerful act of self-care. By saying no to what doesn't serve you, you're saying yes to what matters most. Practice setting boundaries with kindness and firmness, and don't feel guilty for prioritizing your time and energy.

Reflection Question: What rituals can you implement to protect your time? What boundaries do you need to set with yourself or others to ensure your time is spent wisely?

Closing Message: Time is the Ultimate Currency of a Life Well-Lived

As you embark on your journey to master time, remember this: time is the ultimate currency of a life well-lived. Every moment you spend is an investment in your future, and how you choose to spend that time shapes the person you become. By mastering your time, you are not just becoming more efficient — you are becoming more intentional, more aligned with your purpose, and more powerful in your pursuit of greatness.

Time mastery isn't about doing more. It's about living more. Living with passion, with clarity, and with purpose. It's about creating space for the things that truly matter and letting go of the things that no longer serve you. It's about crafting a life that reflects the vision you hold for yourself — a life of meaning, joy, and fulfillment.

You have the power to shape your days, and in doing so, you shape your destiny. Take control of your time, and you will take control of your life. The unstoppable woman in you is waiting to emerge — let time be the fuel that ignites your fire.

9. Navigating Work-Life Balance

Balancing the demands of work and personal life is one of the most complex challenges of modern living. For many women, the pressure to excel in their careers while simultaneously nurturing relationships, family, and personal well-being can feel overwhelming. The pursuit of "having it all" often translates into an exhausting juggling act that leaves little room for self-care or fulfillment. This chapter delves into the nuanced landscape of work-life balance, offering practical, actionable strategies to help you navigate this demanding terrain without compromising your personal goals, well-being, or happiness.

The Myth of Perfect Balance

The first, and perhaps most important, step-in achieving work-life balance is to dispel the myth of perfection. The notion that work and life can coexist in perfect harmony is not only unrealistic but potentially harmful. Balance is not a fixed state of equilibrium; rather, it is dynamic and ever-evolving, shaped by factors such as career demands, family responsibilities, personal health, and societal expectations. Accepting that balance looks different for everyone—and that it fluctuates over time—can relieve the pressure of striving toward an unattainable standard. In reality, balance means making choices that reflect your current priorities and allowing yourself the flexibility to adapt as those priorities shift.

Setting Priorities: Your Compass for Decision-Making

Achieving work-life balance begins with understanding your values and setting clear priorities. What matters most to you? Is it advancing in your career, spending quality time with family, or investing in personal growth? Once you've identified what truly drives you, those priorities can act as your compass, guiding your decisions and helping you allocate your time and energy more effectively. Create a list of your top priorities and regularly refer to it to ensure that your daily actions are in alignment with your long-term goals. This process not only clarifies where you should focus your attention but also empowers you to make conscious decisions that serve your broader aspirations.

Time Management: The Key to Balancing Competing Demands

Effective time management is essential for maintaining a balance between work and personal life. Here are several strategies that can help:

1. **Time Blocking**: Divide your day into dedicated blocks of time for work, family, self-care, and other personal activities. By committing specific hours to each aspect of your life, you minimize distractions and increase focus, reducing the likelihood that work will encroach on personal time.
2. **The 80/20 Rule**: Also known as the Pareto Principle, this rule suggests that 80% of your results come from 20% of your efforts. Identify the tasks that deliver the most significant outcomes and focus your energy on those, rather than trying to accomplish everything at once.
3. **Delegation**: You don't need to do it all yourself. Whether it's at work or home, delegate tasks to others whenever possible. This frees up time and mental space for more meaningful activities.
4. **Saying No**: One of the most powerful tools for achieving balance is learning how to say no. Protect your time by declining tasks and commitments that don't align with your priorities. Saying no is not a weakness — it's an affirmation of your focus on what truly matters.

Embracing Flexibility: The Power of Adaptation

Life is unpredictable, and one of the most important qualities you can cultivate in your pursuit of work-life balance is flexibility. There will be times when work demands more of your attention, and other times when personal matters take precedence. Embrace the ebb and flow of life and be willing to adjust your plans when necessary. Flexibility also means being kind to yourself when things don't go as planned. Instead of striving for perfection, aim for progress. A key to long-term success is the ability to adapt to changing circumstances without losing sight of your ultimate priorities.

Self-Care: The Foundation of Balance

Self-care is often the first casualty in the pursuit of work-life balance, but it is the very foundation upon which sustainable balance rests. When you neglect self-care, your ability to manage both work and personal life deteriorates. Prioritize activities that replenish and rejuvenate you—whether it's exercise, reading, meditation, or simply taking a moment to breathe. Self-care isn't a luxury; it's a necessity. By investing in your well-being, you increase your capacity to handle challenges in all areas of life. Remember, self-care is not selfish; it is an essential act of self-preservation that benefits not only you but also those around you.

Building a Support System: You Don't Have to Do It Alone

The idea that you must manage everything on your own is not only isolating but also unrealistic. Building a strong support system is critical to successfully navigating the challenges of work-life balance. This support can come in many forms:

1. **Family and Friends**: Lean on those closest to you for emotional support, practical assistance, or simply a

listening ear. Asking for help is a sign of strength, not weakness.
2. **Professional Networks**: Foster relationships with colleagues, mentors, and peers who understand your career challenges and can offer guidance, support, or advice.
3. **Community Resources**: Take advantage of community resources such as childcare services, professional coaching, or wellness programs. These services exist to help you manage your responsibilities more effectively.

A strong support network not only alleviates the burden of juggling multiple roles but also provides a sense of solidarity and encouragement.

Creating Boundaries: Defining Your Limits

Establishing and maintaining clear boundaries is essential for achieving a sustainable work-life balance. Boundaries protect your time and energy by delineating where work ends, and personal life begins. This might mean setting specific work hours, turning off email notifications after a certain time, or designating a space in your home that is exclusively for work. Communicating your boundaries clearly to colleagues, family, and friends ensures that they are respected and followed. Boundaries help prevent one aspect of your life from overwhelming the other and allow you to fully engage in each area without feeling stretched too thin.

Redefining Success: Living on Your Terms

Ultimately, achieving work-life balance requires redefining what success means to you. Success doesn't have to mean excelling in every area of life all the time. Instead, it can mean living a life that reflects your values and priorities, where your time and energy are spent on what truly matters. Redefining success also involves permitting yourself to be imperfect, to change course when necessary, and to prioritize your well-being alongside your ambitions. Success is personal, and by focusing on what brings you fulfillment and joy, you can create a more meaningful and balanced life.

Navigating Work-Life Balance as a Woman: Unique Considerations

For many women, the pursuit of work-life balance comes with additional layers of complexity. Women often find themselves juggling multiple roles — whether it's excelling in their careers, managing household responsibilities, or pursuing personal goals. Navigating these roles is both an art and a necessity. Here are some unique challenges women often face:

1. **The Double Shift**: Many women engage in a "double shift" — balancing the demands of their careers while shouldering a significant portion of household responsibilities. Finding strategies to share these responsibilities equitably is crucial.
2. **The Guilt Complex**: Women often struggle with guilt when they prioritize their careers or take time for themselves. Recognizing that self-care is not selfish but necessary for the well-being of both you and your loved ones is a key aspect of achieving balance.
3. **Unrealistic Expectations**: Society often places unrealistic expectations on women, assuming they can effortlessly manage work, family, and personal growth. Overcoming these expectations requires setting boundaries, being realistic about what's achievable, and recognizing that no one can do it all.

Strategies for Thriving

1. **Prioritize Self-Care**: Make self-care a top priority, not an afterthought. A consistent self-care routine will boost

your energy, improve your mental health, and help you better navigate the demands of life.

2. **Master Time Management**: Efficient time management is key to balancing multiple roles. Use tools like calendars and task management apps to streamline your schedule and stay organized.

3. **Set Clear Boundaries**: Protect your time by setting clear boundaries between work and home life. This helps prevent burnout and ensures you have time to recharge.

4. **Seek Support**: Don't hesitate to ask for help. Delegating responsibilities at home or work and seeking assistance from friends, family, or professionals can lighten your load.

5. **Celebrate Successes**: Regularly acknowledge and celebrate your achievements, whether big or small. This practice keeps you motivated and reinforces your commitment to work-life balance.

Self-Reflection & Prioritization:

1. What are your top three priorities in life right now? How do these priorities influence your daily decisions and time allocation?
2. Reflect on a time when you felt your work-life balance was well-managed. What factors contributed to that sense of balance? How can you replicate those factors?
3. How do you currently manage competing demands between your work and personal life? What strategies could help you better navigate these competing demands?

The Myth of Perfect Balance:

4. Do you find yourself striving for a "perfect" balance between work and life? If so, how has this impacted your well-being or productivity?

5. What does work-life balance look like for you at this stage of your life? How has it evolved?

Time Management & Boundaries:

6. What time management strategies have you used to balance your work and personal life? Which ones have worked well, and which haven't?
7. How do you set and maintain boundaries between work and personal time? Can you think of a situation where establishing firmer boundaries could improve your balance?
8. Have you ever felt guilty for saying "no" to work or personal obligations? How did you handle the situation, and what did you learn from it?

Delegation & Support Systems:

9. What tasks or responsibilities in your life could you delegate to others? How could the delegation help you achieve a better balance?
10. Who in your life provides you with the most support, and how could you lean on them more effectively?
11. Are there additional support systems (e.g., childcare, mentorship, professional networks) you could tap into to lighten your load?

Flexibility & Self-Care:

12. How do you handle unexpected changes or disruptions in your schedule? What strategies help you remain flexible while still maintaining your priorities?
13. What are some self-care practices you currently have in place? How do they benefit your mental and physical health? How can you make self-care a non-negotiable part of your routine?

14. Think of a time when you sacrificed self-care for work or other commitments. How did that affect your overall well-being? What can you do to ensure it doesn't happen again?

Redefining Success:

15. How do you define success in your life — both professionally and personally? Do these definitions align with your current work-life balance goals?
16. Are there any societal or internal pressures that make you feel you must "have it all"? How can you shift your mindset to prioritize your unique version of success?

Challenges & Triumphs:

17. Can you recall a specific challenge you've faced in balancing your work and personal life? How did you overcome it, and what did it teach you?
18. Reflect on a recent success — whether personal or professional — that made you feel accomplished. How did that success contribute to your overall sense of balance?

Empowerment Through Balance

Navigating work-life balance is not about achieving perfection, but about finding a rhythm that aligns with your unique values, priorities, and goals. Balance is dynamic and ever-evolving, requiring flexibility, self-awareness, and the courage to set boundaries. Rather than chasing an elusive ideal, it's about making intentional choices that support your well-being and allow you to thrive both personally and professionally.

Ultimately, work-life balance is about giving yourself the permission to redefine success on your own terms. By embracing self-care, prioritizing what truly matters, and seeking support when needed, you can create a life that feels fulfilling and aligned with your aspirations. Balance is not the end goal but a continuous journey — one that evolves as your life changes. The key is to remain adaptable, patient with yourself, and committed to your overall well-being.

Summary of Key Takeaways

- **Work-life balance is dynamic, not static**: It shifts based on life circumstances, so it's important to stay flexible and adjust your expectations as needed.
- **There's no such thing as a perfect balance**: Dispelling the myth of perfection can help reduce pressure and guilt, allowing you to focus on what's truly important to you.
- **Prioritize what matters most**: Clearly define your personal and professional priorities and let them guide your decisions and actions. Regularly reassess and adjust as your goals evolve.
- **Time management is key**: Use strategies like time blocking, the 80/20 rule, and delegation to ensure that your time is used effectively.
- **Set and maintain boundaries**: Protect your personal time by establishing clear boundaries between work and life, and communicate them clearly to others.
- **Self-care is non-negotiable**: Prioritizing your physical, mental, and emotional well-being is essential for maintaining balance and long-term success.
- **Build a support system**: Rely on family, friends, and professional networks for help, guidance, and emotional support as you navigate the demands of work and personal life.
- **Redefine success on your terms**: Success doesn't mean being perfect in all areas of life. It's about aligning your life with your values and finding fulfillment in your own unique journey.

Encouragement for the Journey Ahead

Remember, achieving work-life balance is not a one-time achievement but a lifelong process of self-discovery and adjustment. As you move forward, embrace the fact that balance will look different at different stages of your life. Give yourself the grace to adapt, the strength to prioritize self-care, and the courage to let go of perfection. Your journey is yours to shape—one that is full of opportunities for growth, fulfillment, and success, however you choose to define it.

9. Overcoming Self-Doubt

Self-doubt can feel like an invisible barrier, silently sabotaging our ambitions, dreams, and personal fulfillment. For many women, it's one of the most persistent obstacles to unlocking their full potential. The whisper of "I'm not good enough" can derail progress and diminish confidence. But here's a profound truth: **self-doubt is not a permanent state**. It can be challenged, redefined, and conquered. The journey to overcoming it begins with acknowledging its presence and reclaiming your power.

Overcoming self-doubt is a profound and deeply personal journey, especially for women who face unique challenges and societal expectations. While the road to unwavering confidence may seem daunting, it is entirely achievable. In this chapter, we will explore the intricacies of conquering self-doubt from a woman's perspective, sharing insights, strategies, and stories of triumph to empower you to reclaim your confidence and embrace your potential.

The Roots of Self-Doubt

Before learning how to overcome self-doubt, it's important to understand where it comes from. Often, self-doubt is rooted in societal pressures, past experiences, or deeply ingrained beliefs. From a young age, many women are subjected to limiting stereotypes, cultural expectations, or personal criticism, all of which contribute to feelings of inadequacy.

As we navigate life's challenges, we internalize these voices, creating an **inner critic** that thrives on comparison, perfectionism, and fear. This inner critic is what keeps many women from pursuing their passions or stepping into leadership roles. Yet, here's the key: **self-doubt is not reflective of your abilities**, but a distorted perception of who you truly are.

The Struggles of Self-Doubt

Self-doubt can be a formidable adversary, one that stands in the way of our aspirations, goals, and dreams. For many women, self-doubt is fueled by societal pressures, perfectionism, imposter syndrome, and the constant juggling of roles. Here are some of the common challenges women face on the path to self-confidence:

1. **Imposter Syndrome**: Many women feel like they are not worthy of their accomplishments or fear being exposed as frauds. This persistent sense of inadequacy, despite evident success, can severely undermine self-belief.
2. **Societal Expectations**: From conforming to traditional gender roles to meeting unrealistic beauty standards, societal pressures often contribute to self-doubt, making us feel as though we must constantly meet unattainable expectations.
3. **Balancing Multiple Roles**: The struggle to excel as professionals, caregivers, partners, and more can lead to self-doubt. The weight of feeling that we must do everything perfectly creates overwhelming pressure.
4. **Perfectionism**: The pursuit of perfection often leads to paralyzing self-doubt. When we set impossibly high standards, the fear of failure becomes so intense that we may avoid pursuing our true passions altogether.
5. **Fear of Speaking Up**: Many women hesitate to assert themselves due to a fear of judgment or rejection. This lack of confidence in our voice can lead to self-silencing, eroding our sense of self-worth.

These challenges can feel insurmountable, but they do not define us. The key lies in recognizing these struggles and actively working to dismantle the negative narratives that fuel self-doubt.

Rewriting the Narrative: Strategies for Conquering Self-Doubt

While self-doubt may be persistent, it is far from unbeatable. By recognizing it for what it is and adopting strategies to challenge it, you can reclaim your confidence and unlock your full potential. Below are six powerful steps to help you rise above self-doubt and step boldly into your power.

1. Embrace Imperfection

The pursuit of perfection is one of the greatest sources of self-doubt. Many women are conditioned to believe that they must be flawless to be worthy of success. This myth leads to a constant state of self-criticism. Perfection is unattainable, and striving for it sets you up for disappointment.

Instead, embrace the idea that **imperfection is not only inevitable but necessary for growth**. Mistakes are part of the learning process. Rather than seeing them as failures, recognize them as opportunities to develop resilience and adaptability. When you accept your imperfections, you release the pressure to always get it right, allowing room for growth and progress.

2. Celebrate Your Strengths

Women often focus more on what they haven't achieved, discounting the victories they've already secured. To overcome self-doubt, start by **acknowledging your own achievements**. Take time to list your accomplishments — no matter how small they may seem. Reflect on the challenges you've overcome and the skills you've developed along the way.

Success is often built on incremental progress. By recognizing your past achievements, you reinforce your ability to succeed in the future. Your track record of resilience, adaptability, and strength is evidence that you are more than capable of overcoming whatever lies ahead. **Celebrate your wins—** they're a testament to your ability to navigate adversity.

3. Reframe Your Thoughts

Negative thinking is a core driver of self-doubt. Thoughts like "I can't do this," or "I'm not good enough," create mental barriers that prevent you from taking action. Overcoming self-doubt requires **reframing these thoughts**. Instead of focusing on what you can't do, shift your thinking to what you can learn or how you can improve.

For example, if you catch yourself thinking, "I'm not ready for this opportunity," reframe it to, "I'm prepared to learn and grow in this role." This shift from a fixed mindset to a **growth mindset** allows you to see challenges as opportunities for development. When you change your inner dialogue, you take back control of your narrative.

4. Take Action, even in the Face of Fear

Confidence isn't something you wait for—it's something you build through action. Many people mistakenly believe that they must feel fully confident before taking the next step, but **action is the antidote to fear**. Waiting until you feel confident will only fuel your self-doubt. The key is to take action, even when you're uncertain or afraid.

Break your goals into manageable steps and focus on making progress, no matter how small. Each action, no matter how incremental, builds momentum. As you begin to see progress, your confidence will naturally grow. By consistently taking action, you demonstrate to yourself that you are capable, even in moments of doubt.

5. Surround Yourself with Positive Influences

The company you keep has a profound impact on your self-belief. Negative environments or unsupportive people can magnify self-doubt, while positive, supportive networks can help you rise above it. Surround yourself with people who believe in your potential and encourage you to take risks.

Seek out mentors, peers, or friends who challenge you to grow but also uplift and support you. These are the individuals who can remind you of your worth when your inner critic is the loudest. **Building a network of support** is a crucial step in combating self-doubt. Their belief in you can often serve as the bridge to your own self-belief.

6. Practice Self-Compassion

Many women are their own harshest critics. When we make mistakes or feel uncertain, it's easy to fall into a spiral of self-judgment. But overcoming self-doubt requires that we practice **self-compassion**. This means treating yourself with the same kindness and understanding that you would offer a close friend.

When you stumble, rather than berating yourself, offer words of encouragement: "It's okay to not have all the answers. I'm learning." Self-compassion allows you to recover from setbacks more quickly and with greater resilience. It reminds you that you are a work in progress, and that progress itself is something to be proud of.

Rebuilding Self-Confidence: Strategies for Success

Rebuilding self-confidence is an empowering journey, one that requires intention, practice, and perseverance. Here are strategies to help you regain your inner strength, conquer fears, and silence your inner critic:

1. **Recognize and Challenge Negative Self-Talk**: The first step in overcoming self-doubt is identifying and confronting the negative narratives we tell ourselves. When you catch yourself thinking, "I'm not good enough," challenge that thought. Replace it with a positive affirmation, such as, "I am capable, and I have the skills to succeed."
2. **Embrace Self-Care**: Self-care is essential in nurturing your self-esteem. Prioritizing your mental, emotional, and physical well-being provides a strong foundation for confidence. Whether it's through exercise, meditation, journaling, or simply taking time for yourself, self-care reminds you that you are worth the effort.
3. **Set Realistic Goals**: Break down your larger aspirations into achievable, bite-sized goals. Each time you accomplish a goal, no matter how small, it reinforces your belief in your capabilities. Success is cumulative, and progress builds confidence.
4. **Seek Support and Mentorship**: Surrounding yourself with a supportive network can make all the difference. Seek out mentors or peers who believe in your potential and offer guidance. Having people in your corner who lift you up will help bolster your self-belief.
5. **Practice Assertiveness**: Learning to assert yourself — whether by speaking up in meetings, setting boundaries, or advocating for yourself — is key to building self-confidence. Assertiveness allows you to stand in your truth and honor your worth.

6. **Celebrate Achievements**: Take the time to acknowledge your accomplishments. No win is too small. By celebrating your successes, you reinforce your self-worth and cultivate motivation to continue striving toward your goals.

7. **Embrace Vulnerability and Authenticity**: Confidence doesn't mean always being perfect. It means allowing yourself to be vulnerable and authentic. Share your challenges and fears with trusted friends or mentors. Being open fosters deeper connections and reminds you that you are not alone in your journey.

8. **Continuous Learning and Growth**: Life is a continuous process of learning and evolving. By adopting a growth mindset and embracing new opportunities, you expand your capabilities and strengthen your self-confidence with every new experience.

The Power of Resilience: Turning Setbacks into Strength

Resilience is a powerful ally in overcoming self-doubt. Every setback you encounter is an opportunity to develop resilience, a skill that helps you bounce back stronger after each challenge. When faced with obstacles, remind yourself that **your worth is not measured by one failure or one mistake**, but by your ability to get up and keep going.

The road to success is rarely linear, and the most successful women are those who have learned to rise after falling. Resilience allows you to view setbacks not as final destinations, but as detours on your path to growth. Each time you rise after a fall, you reinforce the belief that you are capable of facing whatever comes your way.

Resilience and Empowerment

At the heart of overcoming self-doubt is resilience — the ability to rise after every fall, to learn from setbacks, and to use challenges as steppingstones toward success. Women who have triumphed over self-doubt have embraced resilience as their ally. They've discovered that setbacks do not define them; their ability to persevere does.

Take, for example, the women who have confronted imposter syndrome. They found the courage to acknowledge their fears, then actively sought to dismantle the idea that their success was mere luck. By recognizing their strengths and affirming their achievements, they moved forward with renewed confidence.

Similarly, countless women have defied societal expectations by unapologetically pursuing nontraditional careers or rejecting unrealistic beauty standards. These women didn't allow external pressures to dictate their worth. Instead, they set their own terms and reshaped their lives according to their values.

Turn Doubt into Motivation

What if instead of seeing self-doubt as a barrier, you used it as fuel? Doubt often signals where our deepest fears lie, and where there is fear, there is opportunity for growth. Reframe your doubt as a challenge to overcome, a reason to push yourself even further. Each time you confront your fears, you step closer to realizing your full potential.

What if instead of seeing self-doubt as something to overcome, you used it as fuel for action? Doubt, when reframed, can be a powerful motivator. It shows you where your fears lie and highlights the areas where you want to grow. **Use that awareness to drive you forward.**

Ask yourself, "What am I afraid of, and how can I turn that fear into a challenge to conquer?" By seeing doubt as a signal for where you need to push harder, you can transform it into *an* inner fire that drives you toward your goals. This mindset shift turns doubt from a barrier into a catalyst for action.

For instance, the fear of rejection can often hold us back from taking bold steps, but by facing it head-on, we reclaim our power. Women who have leaned into this discomfort have experienced tremendous personal and professional growth.

The Power of Affirmations and Visualization

Affirmations and visualization are transformative tools for overcoming self-doubt. When you repeat empowering statements like, "I am capable," "I trust myself," or "I deserve success," you begin to reshape your internal narrative. These affirmations help counter the negative self-talk that fuels self-doubt.

Similarly, visualization is a powerful way to combat doubt. **Picture yourself succeeding**—envision the steps, the journey, and the outcome. When your mind becomes familiar with success, it starts to see it as a possibility rather than a distant dream. Visualization primes your brain for action and reinforces the belief that you are capable of achieving your goals.

Celebrating Achievements and Triumphs

One of the most powerful ways to overcome self-doubt is to celebrate your victories, no matter how small they seem. Every achievement is a reminder of your capability and strength. Whether you land a new job, set boundaries in a relationship, or simply take time for self-care, each success reinforces your self-worth.

In addition to your celebrations, it's crucial to recognize the success stories of other women who have triumphed over self-doubt. Their perseverance, resilience, and determination serve as a source of inspiration for us all.

Take the example of women who have embraced their vulnerability, sharing their fears and stories with others. By doing so, they not only strengthened their self-confidence but also empowered others to do the same.

Maintaining Unshakable Confidence

Achieving self-confidence is one part of the journey — maintaining it is another. This requires ongoing effort and mindfulness. Here are habits to help you maintain your self-confidence as you continue to grow:

1. **Continual Self-Reflection**: Regularly assess your strengths and areas for growth. Self-awareness is the foundation for sustained confidence.
2. **Resilience Building**: Embrace challenges as opportunities for growth. Setbacks are part of life, but resilience enables you to bounce back stronger and more confident.
3. **Positive Self-Talk**: Combat self-doubt by maintaining a positive internal dialogue. Affirm your worth and capabilities regularly to reinforce your belief in yourself.
4. **Gratitude and Celebration**: Make it a habit to express gratitude for your accomplishments, no matter how small. Celebrate them to keep your motivation and confidence strong.

Real Women, Real Triumphs: Stories of Overcoming Doubt

Countless women who have achieved extraordinary success have faced their battles with self-doubt. Take **Oprah Winfrey**, for example. Despite her immense success, she has spoken openly about her struggles with feelings of inadequacy. Oprah learned to quiet her inner critic by focusing on her strengths and staying aligned with her purpose.

Similarly, **Serena Williams**, one of the greatest athletes of all time, has shared how self-doubt sometimes crept into her mind throughout her career. Instead of letting it stop her, she channeled that energy into honing her skills and continuously striving for improvement. These women didn't let self-doubt define them — they used it as fuel to rise higher.

Reflective Questions:

1. Which of the common challenges of self-doubt resonates most with your personal experience? How has it affected your confidence?

2. Have you ever experienced imposter syndrome? If so, how did it manifest in your life, and what steps can you take to confront it moving forward?

3. What societal expectations have contributed to your self-doubt? How can you begin to challenge and redefine those expectations in your life?

4. In what areas of your life do you strive for perfection? How has this pursuit of perfection affected your self-confidence and willingness to take risks?

5. Think of a recent achievement, big or small. Did you take the time to celebrate it? How can you make celebration a regular practice to reinforce your self-worth?

6. Who are the people in your life who support and encourage you? How can you further cultivate a network of mentors and like-minded individuals to help you build your confidence?

7. What negative self-talk do you often catch yourself engaging in? How can you begin to replace these thoughts with positive affirmations?

8. How do you prioritize self-care in your daily life? What specific actions can you take to improve your physical, emotional, or mental well-being?

9. In what situations do you find it difficult to assert yourself? How can you practice assertiveness to align your actions with your values and beliefs?

10. How can you reframe your self-doubt as an opportunity for growth rather than an obstacle? Think of a time when facing your fears led to personal or professional progress.

11. How can vulnerability and authenticity enhance your confidence? Is there an area of your life where you're holding back for fear of judgment or rejection?

12. What daily or weekly practices can you implement to maintain and grow your self-confidence? How can continual learning and self-reflection become part of your routine?

13. In moments of self-doubt, what strategies from this chapter can you turn to to regain confidence and stay on track with your goals?

14. Which stories or examples from the chapter inspired you the most? How can you apply those lessons to your own journey of overcoming self-doubt?

15. What is one fear or self-limiting belief that you are committed to facing head-on after reading this chapter? What steps will you take to confront it?

Embracing Your Inner Fire

Your journey to overcoming self-doubt is unique, but you are not alone. Every step you take toward building your confidence is an act of courage and empowerment. By implementing these strategies, nurturing your resilience, and celebrating your successes, you will unlock the unstoppable woman within you

Ultimately, overcoming self-doubt is about more than quieting your inner critic; it's about **embracing your inner fire** — the core of strength, resilience, and potential that exists within every woman. Self-doubt may never completely disappear, but with the right tools and mindset, it will no longer have the power to hold you back.

Every time you take action in the face of fear, every time you reframe a negative thought, and every time you celebrate your progress, you ignite that inner fire. This fire fuels your journey toward becoming the unstoppable woman you were always meant to be. Remember, confidence is not a destination but an ongoing process of growth.

Remember, you are enough. You are capable. You are unstoppable.

Embracing Your Journey Beyond Self-Doubt

Overcoming self-doubt is not a one-time achievement; it's an ongoing journey of self-discovery, growth, and empowerment. In this chapter, we've explored the unique challenges women face in battling self-doubt, from imposter syndrome to societal expectations, perfectionism, and the fear of asserting ourselves. But as we've seen, these obstacles do not define us. By recognizing our struggles and actively taking steps to rebuild our self-confidence, we unlock the power within to shape our lives on our terms.

The key strategies outlined — challenging negative self-talk, embracing self-care, setting realistic goals, seeking support, practicing assertiveness, and celebrating achievements — are not just tools to overcome self-doubt but essential habits for maintaining unshakable confidence in the long term. Each small victory along the way reinforces our strength and capability, reminding us that we are worthy of success, happiness, and fulfillment.

Resilience, perseverance, and vulnerability are the cornerstones of this journey. Every challenge presents an opportunity to grow, and every setback is a steppingstone to greater self-assurance. The women who have triumphed over self-doubt have done so by embracing their authentic selves and refusing to let fear or external pressures hold them back.

As you continue your journey, remember that building self-confidence is a process that requires patience and practice. Each step you take, no matter how small, is a step closer to becoming the unstoppable woman you are meant to be. Trust in your abilities, celebrate your progress, and know that you possess the inner strength to overcome any doubts that come your way.

Your journey of self-discovery is unique, and your confidence will continue to evolve as you grow. Keep moving forward with courage, resilience, and a deep belief in your potential. You are more powerful than your doubts, and by embracing your fire, you can achieve anything you set your heart and mind to. Stay committed, stay strong, and always remember — you are unstoppable.

10. Unlocking Your Inner Creativity

Embrace Your Creative Essence

Creativity is not just a trait; it's a powerful force that fuels innovation, problem-solving, and personal growth. For unstoppable women embracing their fire, tapping into this wellspring of creativity can amplify your impact, both personally and professionally. Here's how you can unlock and harness your creative potential:

1. Embrace Curiosity and Exploration

- Curiosity is the spark that ignites creativity. Foster a mindset of exploration and openness to new ideas. Allow yourself to ask questions and seek out diverse perspectives. Remember, creativity thrives in the realm of the unknown.

2. Cultivate a Creative Routine

- Establishing a routine that nurtures your creativity is essential. Whether it's journaling, sketching, or brainstorming, carve out dedicated time for creative pursuits. Consistency breeds creativity and helps you develop a deeper connection with your creative instincts.

3. Challenge Your Comfort Zone

- Growth often happens outside of your comfort zone. Push yourself to try new techniques, take on unfamiliar tasks, or explore different mediums of expression.

Embracing discomfort fosters resilience and expands your creative boundaries.

4. Collaborate and Seek Feedback

- Collaboration can be a catalyst for innovation. Engage with diverse voices and perspectives to enrich your creative process. Don't shy away from constructive feedback; it's a valuable tool for refining your ideas and enhancing your creative output.

5. Harness Inspiration from Within and Beyond

- Draw inspiration from your life experiences, passions, and the world around you. Explore art, literature, nature, and cultures to ignite fresh ideas. Embrace moments of reflection and solitude to tap into your inner creative reservoir.

6. Embody Fearlessness in Creation

- Creativity flourishes in an environment free from fear of judgment or failure. Embrace the courage to experiment, make mistakes, and learn from them. Trust in your abilities and the unique perspective you bring to every creative endeavor.

7. Celebrate Your Creative Journey

- Recognize and celebrate every milestone, no matter how small. Your creative journey is a testament to your growth and resilience. Share your successes, inspire others, and continue to evolve as fearless creators.

By nurturing your creativity, you not only enrich your own life but also create ripple effects of inspiration and empowerment in the world around you. Embrace your creative fire and let it fuel your path to greatness.

The Creative Journey: Embracing Your Inner Power

Creativity is a powerful force that resides within each of us. It is the wellspring of innovation, fulfillment, and self-expression. Yet, for many women, cultural expectations, self-doubt, and societal pressures can obscure this innate potential. Unleashing your creativity requires courage, determination, and the ability to break free from the constraints holding you back.

Here are some of the challenges women often face on their creative journeys:

1. **Cultural Expectations**: Society often imposes limiting gender roles, discouraging women from pursuing artistic or unconventional endeavors.
2. **Self-Doubt**: Many women grapple with self-doubt, questioning the value of their ideas or hesitating to share them with the world.
3. **Balancing Responsibilities**: Managing creative pursuits alongside work, family, and other responsibilities can seem daunting, leaving little time or energy for self-expression.
4. **Fear of Judgment**: Fear of criticism or not living up to societal expectations can stifle creativity, making women hesitant to take risks.
5. **Perfectionism**: The pressure to meet impossibly high standards can hinder creative expression, leading to self-censorship and a reluctance to experiment.

Strategies for Unleashing Creativity

Despite these challenges, every woman can tap into her creative power. By embracing practical strategies, you can nurture your creativity, overcome self-doubt, and boldly express yourself. Here are key steps to unlocking your creative potential:

1. **Recognize Your Creative Voice**: Start by acknowledging your unique perspective. Your voice is valuable, and your creativity deserves to be expressed. By embracing your authenticity, you open the door to limitless creative possibilities.

2. **Practice Self-Compassion**: Creativity requires vulnerability. Be kind to yourself, especially when faced with self-doubt. Allow yourself to make mistakes and experiment without fear of judgment. Self-compassion is the key to resilience and creative growth.

3. **Prioritize Creative Time**: Make creativity a non-negotiable part of your routine. Set aside dedicated time for creative pursuits, just as you would for any other important responsibility. Guard this time fiercely—it is an investment in your self-expression and well-being.

4. **Learn from Criticism**: Embrace feedback as a tool for growth. Constructive criticism can refine your skills and help you evolve as a creator. Rather than fearing judgment, view it as an opportunity to push your work to new heights.

5. **Collaborate and Build Support Networks**: Surround yourself with like-minded individuals who nurture your creativity. Collaboration and support from others can inspire fresh ideas, bolster your confidence, and fuel your creative momentum.

6. **Release Perfectionism**: Let go of the need for perfection. Creativity is about expression, not flawlessness. Embrace imperfections as part of the process—they often lead to the most innovative outcomes.

Triumph Over Creative Challenges

As women, overcoming creative challenges is not only possible but deeply empowering. Here's how you can triumph over the obstacles in your path:

1. **Embrace Your Unique Voice**: Recognize the value of your perspective. Women who break free from cultural expectations and self-doubt often find strength by embracing their individuality. Your creative voice is powerful — use it boldly.
2. **Build Resilience**: Resilience is essential for overcoming setbacks. Successful women have learned to turn self-doubt, criticism, and failure into steppingstones for growth. Every challenge is an opportunity to build creative strength.
3. **Prioritize Creativity**: Women who triumph in their creative endeavors make time for their passions. They protect their creative time and see it as essential for their well-being and personal fulfillment.
4. **Learn from Setbacks**: Instead of fearing criticism, embrace it. Feedback can sharpen your skills and elevate your work. Creative women see constructive critique as a chance to grow and innovate.

Strategies for Cultivating Creativity

Once you've unlocked your creativity, the next step is to continually nurture and expand it. These strategies will help you maintain and deepen your creative potential:

1. **Creative Rituals**: Establish consistent creative practices. Dedicate time each day or week to writing, painting, dancing, or whatever form of expression speaks to you.
2. **Mindfulness Practices**: Use mindfulness techniques, such as meditation or deep breathing, to calm self-doubt and tap into your inner creative flow.

3. **Creative Prompts**: Sometimes, all it takes is a spark. Creative prompts or challenges can ignite your imagination and help overcome creative blockages.

4. **Explore New Art Forms**: Don't limit yourself to one creative outlet. Experiment with different mediums, from music to dance to visual arts. Exploring new forms can invigorate your creative spirit.

5. **Seek Inspiration Everywhere**: Look to the world around you for inspiration. Nature, art, literature, and everyday life can all provide fresh perspectives and ideas.

6. **Celebrate Creative Milestones**: Acknowledge and celebrate every creative achievement, no matter how small. This builds confidence and reinforces your commitment to creativity.

Triumph Over Creative Challenges

As women, overcoming creative challenges is not only possible but deeply empowering. Here's how you can triumph over the obstacles in your path:

1. **Embrace Your Unique Voice**: Recognize the value of your perspective. Women who break free from cultural expectations and self-doubt often find strength by embracing their individuality. Your creative voice is powerful—use it boldly.

2. **Build Resilience**: Resilience is essential for overcoming setbacks. Successful women have learned to turn self-doubt, criticism, and failure into steppingstones for growth. Every challenge is an opportunity to build creative strength.

3. **Prioritize Creativity**: Women who triumph in their creative endeavors make time for their passions. They protect their creative time and see it as essential for their well-being and personal fulfillment.

4. **Learn from Setbacks**: Instead of fearing criticism, embrace it. Feedback can sharpen your skills and elevate your work. Creative women see constructive critique as a chance to grow and innovate.

Strategies for Cultivating Creativity

Once you've unlocked your creativity, the next step is to continually nurture and expand it. These strategies will help you maintain and deepen your creative potential:

1. **Creative Rituals**: Establish consistent creative practices. Dedicate time each day or week to writing, painting, dancing, or whatever form of expression speaks to you.
2. **Mindfulness Practices**: Use mindfulness techniques, such as meditation or deep breathing, to calm self-doubt and tap into your inner creative flow.
3. **Creative Prompts**: Sometimes, all it takes is a spark. Creative prompts or challenges can ignite your imagination and help overcome creative blockages.
4. **Explore New Art Forms**: Don't limit yourself to one creative outlet. Experiment with different mediums, from music to dance to visual arts. Exploring new forms can invigorate your creative spirit.
5. **Seek Inspiration Everywhere**: Look to the world around you for inspiration. Nature, art, literature, and everyday life can all provide fresh perspectives and ideas.
6. **Celebrate Creative Milestones**: Acknowledge and celebrate every creative achievement, no matter how small. This builds confidence and reinforces your commitment to creativity.

The Power of Creativity for Unstoppable Women

Creativity is not just a trait—it's a life force, a key to unlocking new possibilities, both within ourselves and in the world around us. For unstoppable women who are embracing their fire, creativity is the bridge between vision and action. It fuels innovation, cultivates resilience, and becomes a driving force that can take you from ordinary to extraordinary.

Being creative is not reserved for artists or musicians; it is a fundamental skill for all women who seek to make an impact. Whether you're navigating your career, solving problems, or building meaningful relationships, creativity is your ally. It empowers you to think beyond the obvious, to take risks, and to step into your most authentic, empowered self.

Here's how you can unlock your creative potential and allow it to fuel your journey as an unstoppable woman embracing her fire.

1. Ignite Your Curiosity

Creativity begins with curiosity. It's about asking, "What if?" — and then fearlessly pursuing the answer. Embrace a mindset of exploration and allow yourself to be open to new ideas, experiences, and perspectives. The more curious you are, the more innovative you become.

Never stop learning. Seek out diverse sources of inspiration, whether through books, conversations with different people, or immersing yourself in unfamiliar environments. Creativity thrives in diversity — of thought, experience, and challenge.

2. Design a Creative Routine

Creativity isn't random; it's cultivated. Like any skill, it grows with consistent practice. Designing a routine that encourages creative thinking is essential for building this capacity. Dedicate time each day to reflect, journal, brainstorm, or engage in activities that stimulate your mind.

Remember, consistency builds momentum. Just as muscles grow stronger with regular exercise, your creativity expands with regular attention. The more often you engage with your creative side, the easier it becomes to tap into it.

3. Step Outside Your Comfort Zone

Great things happen when we push ourselves beyond the familiar. Creativity requires us to take risks, embrace discomfort, and challenge what we know. As an unstoppable woman, you must be willing to step into the unknown, try new things, and face potential failure head-on.

Whether it's learning a new skill, exploring different methods to solve a problem, or taking on unfamiliar projects, this willingness to experiment will not only sharpen your creative instincts but also strengthen your resilience. Failure isn't the end—it's a lesson that can lead to your next breakthrough.

4. Collaborate and Connect

Creativity flourishes in collaboration. Engaging with others—especially those from different backgrounds or fields—can spark fresh ideas and solutions you may never have considered on your own. Collaboration brings new energy, challenges your thinking, and pushes you to expand beyond your mental boundaries.

Seek feedback from trusted sources who can offer constructive critique. A key part of the creative process is refining your ideas, and this refinement often comes through dialogue. By connecting with others, you gain access to insights that enhance your creative vision.

5. Find Inspiration Everywhere

Creativity is all around you — if you're willing to see it. Whether in nature, art, music, or even the patterns of everyday life, inspiration is abundant. Take time to immerse yourself in activities and environments that stimulate your senses. Let the beauty and complexity of the world ignite your creative fire.

At the same time, look within. Your personal experiences, challenges, and triumphs are a rich source of creativity. Don't be afraid to draw from your own story—it's unique and powerful, and it can inspire not just you, but others as well.

6. Embrace Imperfection and Fearlessness

The greatest obstacle to creativity is the fear of being wrong or imperfect. Yet, true creativity comes from a place of fearlessness. You must permit yourself to create without judgment, to make mistakes, and to see those mistakes as steppingstones to greatness.

Embracing imperfection is a crucial part of the creative process. It's in those messy, uncertain moments that true breakthroughs occur. Trust in your ability to navigate the unknown and remember that the act of creating itself is where the magic happens — not just in the final product.

7. Celebrate the Journey, Not Just the Destination

Unlocking your creativity is a continuous journey, not a destination. It's an evolving process, one that requires patience, persistence, and celebration. Every small creative victory counts. Celebrate your progress, even the smallest achievements, and use them as motivation to keep moving forward.

As an unstoppable woman, your creative journey is an expression of your strength, courage, and uniqueness. By embracing this journey, you not only empower yourself but also inspire those around you.

The Importance of Self-Care

To sustain creativity, you must take care of yourself — physically, emotionally, and mentally. Prioritizing self-care helps maintain your energy, focus, and passion. Adequate rest, exercise, and time for reflection are vital for nourishing your creative soul.

Celebrating Your Creative Journey

Unlocking and nurturing creativity is an empowering journey. It's not just about the finished product — it's about the process of discovering your voice, overcoming challenges, and daring to express yourself fully. Every step, every attempt, and every creation is a testament to your resilience, courage, and commitment to self-expression.

Remember, your creative journey is unique. By embracing your creativity, you not only enrich your own life but also inspire others to embark on their journeys of self-expression. Unleashing your creativity is a transformative, ongoing process — one that contributes to your personal growth, confidence, and overall well-being.

As a woman embracing her fire, let your creativity guide you. It's time to step into your power, unleash your potential, and share your brilliance with the world.

1. Recognizing Your Unique Creative Voice:

- What are some creative pursuits or ideas that excite you, but you've been hesitant to explore?
- How do you think your personal experiences and perspective influence your creativity?

2. Overcoming Challenges:

- What societal expectations or internal doubts have held you back from embracing your creativity?
- Reflect on a time when fear of judgment or perfectionism stopped you from completing a creative project. What could you have done differently?

3. Time for Creativity:

- How much time do you currently dedicate to creative activities each week? What small changes could you make to prioritize this time more effectively?
- Think about your daily routine. What moments in your schedule could be repurposed for creative exploration?

4. Embracing Imperfection:

- Can you identify an area of your life where perfectionism has limited your creative freedom? How can you begin to let go of the need for perfection?
- What would happen if you allowed yourself to create freely without worrying about the outcome? How would that feel?

5. Creative Experimentation:

- What is one creative activity or medium you've never tried but are curious about? How could experimenting with it unlock new inspiration?
- If you were to explore a new creative outlet this week, what would it be, and why?

6. Seeking Support:

- Do you have a network of supportive, creative peers? If not, where could you find or build a community that encourages your artistic growth?

- Who in your life could you collaborate with on a creative project? What kind of project would it be?

7. Mindfulness and Creativity:

- How do you currently handle moments of creative block or self-doubt? Could mindfulness practices like meditation or journaling help you unlock new ideas?
- Next time you feel stuck creatively, try pausing and taking deep breaths. What immediate changes do you notice in your thinking or energy?

8. Reflection and Resilience:

- Think of a time when you experienced a creative failure. What lessons did you learn, and how did it shape your resilience for future projects?
- How can you reframe failures as opportunities for growth rather than setbacks?

9. Celebrating Your Creative Journey:

- What creative milestone, no matter how small, are you most proud of? How can you celebrate this achievement?
- What creative goal would you like to set for yourself for the next month, and how will you hold yourself accountable to achieve it?

10. Leadership and Creativity:

- In what areas of your life do you see yourself as a leader? How could embracing your creativity make you a more innovative and impactful leader?
- Think of a challenge you're facing in your work or personal life. How could approaching it with creativity help you find a solution?

Embrace Your Creative Power

Unlocking your creativity is more than an artistic pursuit — it is a journey of self-discovery, empowerment, and personal growth. As we've explored in this chapter, women often face unique challenges on their creative path, from societal expectations and self-doubt to the pressure of perfectionism. However, by recognizing these obstacles and developing practical strategies to overcome them, you can unleash your full creative potential.

Remember, creativity is not limited to any one medium or form. It is found in how you solve problems, approach challenges, and express your ideas. By prioritizing time for creativity, embracing imperfection, seeking support, and learning from criticism, you begin to cultivate a mindset of innovation and self-expression.

Your creative voice is unique, and it deserves to be heard. Whether through painting, writing, dance, or any other form of expression, your contributions are valuable and impactful. As you progress on this journey, continue to celebrate both small and large victories, and remain resilient in the face of challenges.

Creativity is a lifelong journey. As you unlock your creative fire, remember that it's a continually evolving process. Every new experience, challenge, and experiment will only deepen your understanding of yourself and your creative abilities.

So, keep going. Continue exploring, experimenting, and expressing your unique perspective. Embrace the unknown, trust your instincts, and most importantly, honor your creativity. As an unstoppable woman, you have the power to shape not only your own life but also the world around you with the limitless potential of your creative fire.

This is your moment—embrace it and let your creativity soar.

11. BUILDING YOUR CREATIVITY

Building Creativity and Nurturing Healthy Relationships

In the journey of becoming an unstoppable woman, creativity and relationships are two pivotal forces that shape not only how we engage with the world, but also how we view ourselves. Both are deeply intertwined and essential for personal growth, emotional well-being, and empowerment. We will explore how embracing creativity can elevate our ability to build and maintain healthy relationships, and how fostering meaningful connections enriches our creative potential. Together, these practices empower women to thrive in every aspect of life. In the journey of becoming an unstoppable woman, two powerful forces, creativity and relationships, shape how we engage with the world and evolve as individuals. Creativity enables us to view the world with fresh eyes, while healthy relationships provide the emotional foundation for growth, support, and self-realization. When combined, these elements create a dynamic synergy that empowers women to thrive in all aspects of life.

This chapter explores how nurturing creativity can strengthen your relationships, and in turn, how fostering meaningful connections can unlock your creative potential. By embracing both, you can elevate your emotional well-being, confidence, and overall life satisfaction.

The Power of Creativity in Building Relationships

Creativity is more than an artistic skill — it is a mindset that allows us to think outside the box, solve problems, and communicate more effectively. When we embrace our creative selves, we open up new possibilities for building connections, whether it's with friends, family, or romantic partners. Creativity helps us navigate the complexities of relationships by encouraging empathy, innovation, and adaptability.

For women, creativity often plays an unspoken role in how we form and nurture relationships. Whether it's through problem-solving in a challenging conversation or finding new ways to support and uplift others, creativity allows us to cultivate deeper, more meaningful connections. When you embrace your inner creativity, you not only enrich your personal life but also positively impact the lives of those around you.

The Importance of Healthy Relationships

Healthy relationships are the foundation of a fulfilling life. As women, we often place a strong emphasis on our connections with others, and these relationships can significantly influence our emotional and mental well-being. They provide support, understanding, and a sense of belonging. However, societal expectations and personal pressures can sometimes make maintaining these relationships challenging. It is essential to understand the importance of healthy relationships and to approach them with creativity and intentionality.

Healthy relationships require balance, communication, and mutual respect, but they also need adaptability—a key aspect of creativity. Being able to adjust your approach, find innovative ways to maintain emotional intimacy, or resolve conflicts is crucial to nurturing connections that last. Creativity allows you to see your relationships from new angles, offering solutions to challenges and enhancing your bonds.

Scientific Backing: How Creativity Enhances Relationships

Numerous studies show that creativity and emotional intelligence go hand in hand. Creative problem-solving enhances empathy and emotional awareness, both of which are critical for building strong relationships.

- **Creativity and Empathy:** Research has shown that engaging in creative activities—whether it's art, writing, or even creative thinking—stimulates the brain's empathy centers. The ability to think imaginatively allows us to put ourselves in another person's shoes, fostering deeper emotional connections.

- **Creative Problem-Solving Reduces Stress:** Relationships often face tension, but creativity helps mitigate stress by offering new, less confrontational ways to approach issues. Creative conflict resolution leads to less emotional reactivity and more thoughtful, constructive conversations.

The Challenges Women Face in Building Relationships

Women often face unique challenges when it comes to building and maintaining relationships. Societal norms, cultural expectations, and the constant juggling of multiple roles—caregiver, professional, friend—can make this journey even more complex. However, by infusing creativity into how we approach these hurdles, we can transform challenges into opportunities for growth.

1. **Societal Expectations:** Women are frequently expected to be nurturing, supportive, and accommodating in their relationships. These expectations can hinder open communication and self-expression, making it difficult to assert personal needs and desires.
2. **Balancing Multiple Roles:** Juggling roles as caregivers, professionals, and partners can be overwhelming, leaving little time for self-care or personal relationships. Striking a balance between your responsibilities and relationships often requires creative thinking and innovative time management.
3. **Communication Barriers:** Women may face communication barriers due to fear of confrontation or cultural norms that discourage assertiveness. Learning to communicate openly and assertively is key to building and maintaining healthy connections.

4. **Self-Care Neglect:** Prioritizing self-care can be a challenge for women who often put others' needs before their own. Yet, without self-care, it becomes difficult to sustain healthy relationships. Creative self-care practices can ensure that you have the emotional bandwidth to nurture others.

5. **Empowerment and Boundaries:** Establishing healthy boundaries is essential, but many women struggle with fear of being perceived as demanding or assertive. Creativity in setting boundaries can help you assert your needs while maintaining positive, respectful relationships.

Practical Exercises to Boost Creativity in Relationships

Here are some practical exercises designed to strengthen both creativity and relationships:

- **Creative Journaling:** Set aside 15 minutes each day to write about your relationships. Use prompts such as, "What is one creative way I can show appreciation to someone I love today?" or "How can I approach a current challenge in my relationship differently?"
- **Vision Board for Relationships:** Create a visual representation of what healthy relationships look like to you. Use images, words, and symbols to inspire new ways of approaching the people in your life.
- **Art Therapy for Emotional Expression:** When dealing with a difficult relationship, take a break from verbal communication and engage in creative expression. Draw or paint how you feel, then use that artwork as a conversation starter to communicate your emotions.

Affirmations for Creativity and Healthy Relationships

Affirmations can serve as empowering reminders of your capacity to build meaningful connections through creativity:

- "I nurture my creativity to build deeper, more authentic relationships."
- "My relationships are grounded in mutual respect, understanding, and growth."
- "I have the power to creatively resolve conflicts and strengthen my connections."
- "By expressing myself creatively, I invite joy and fulfillment into my relationships."

Embracing Vulnerability and Authenticity

Creativity often demands vulnerability. Just as in art, where we expose our innermost thoughts and feelings, building healthy relationships requires us to be authentic and open. Vulnerability may feel risky, but it creates space for genuine connection.

- **Vulnerability in Creativity:** Allow yourself to experiment, take risks, and embrace imperfections in your creative endeavors. Doing so fosters emotional resilience, which is essential for deep, trusting relationships.
- **Authenticity in Relationships:** Healthy relationships thrive on authenticity. When you are true to yourself, you allow others to connect with the real you. Creativity helps you express your unique personality and values, ensuring that your relationships are built on honesty and trust.

Strategies for Building Healthy Relationships Through Creativity

To build and maintain healthy relationships, creativity can be your greatest asset. Here are key strategies that incorporate creativity into your approach:

1. **Cultivate Self-Awareness:** Self-awareness is the foundation of all healthy relationships. Get creative in how you explore your inner world—journaling, meditation, or expressive arts can help you understand your needs, values, and boundaries.
2. **Communicate Effectively:** Creativity in communication means finding new ways to express your thoughts and emotions. Whether it's through words, actions, or even silence, explore various forms of communication to connect with others.
3. **Set and Maintain Boundaries:** Setting boundaries doesn't always mean saying "no." It can involve creative compromises or finding alternative ways to meet everyone's needs without sacrificing your well-being.
4. **Empowerment through Expression:** Embrace empowerment by learning to express your needs in ways that feel authentic to you. Creative expression—whether through art, writing, or other mediums—can help you assert yourself confidently.
5. **Build a Supportive Network:** Creative problem-solving in relationships includes seeking support when needed. Whether it's a heart-to-heart with a trusted friend or joining a community group, engaging with others can provide new perspectives and solutions to relationship challenges.
6. **Resolve Conflict Creatively:** Conflict is inevitable in any relationship, but creativity can help resolve it constructively. Explore different ways to understand and approach disagreements—perhaps through role-playing, open-ended questions, or taking a break to reflect on the situation.
7. **Celebrate Milestones Creatively:** Whether it's celebrating anniversaries, personal achievements, or simply expressing gratitude, find creative ways to celebrate the milestones in your relationships. It strengthens the emotional bond and affirms your commitment to the connection.

Empowerment through Creativity and Healthy Relationships

Creativity and relationships have a symbiotic relationship. As you cultivate creativity, you naturally become more adaptable, empathetic, and solution-oriented—qualities that enhance your relationships. On the other hand, as you nurture healthy connections, you gain emotional strength and inspiration, which fuels your creative pursuits.

For example, a woman who feels supported in her relationships is more likely to take creative risks, whether in her career or personal life. Similarly, a woman who regularly exercises her creativity through art, writing, or problem-solving is more likely to approach relationships with curiosity and a growth mindset. The two feed into one another, creating a cycle of empowerment and fulfillment.

The Role of Self-Care in Creativity and Relationships

Self-care is vital for nurturing both creativity and relationships. When we neglect our well-being, it becomes difficult to maintain our energy, focus, and emotional balance. Creativity can also play a key role in self-care. Engaging in creative activities—whether it's painting, cooking, gardening, or writing—can rejuvenate your spirit, providing the emotional resilience needed to invest in relationships.

Additionally, practicing self-care encourages a stronger sense of self, which is crucial for setting healthy boundaries and maintaining balanced relationships. When you are emotionally and physically well, you are better equipped to nurture others.

The Role of Self-Care in Creativity and Relationships

Self-care is vital for nurturing creativity and relationships alike. Without taking time to recharge, it's difficult to maintain the energy needed for meaningful connections. Creative self-care practices can help keep your emotional and mental well-being intact.

- **Creative Self-Care Ideas:** Try activities like journaling, painting, dancing, or even cooking as ways to both nurture yourself and tap into your creativity. These moments of self-expression refresh your spirit, allowing you to approach your relationships with renewed energy.

Call to Action: Take Your Creativity and Relationships to the Next Level

This is your time to embrace creativity as a tool to strengthen your relationships and empower your personal growth. Challenge yourself to take small steps that bring both creativity and connection into your daily life.

- **30-Minute Creativity Challenge:** Set aside 30 minutes each week to engage in a creative activity—whether it's writing, painting, or problem-solving—that nurtures your soul. Reflect on how this practice enhances your relationships.
- **Creative Connection Challenge:** Reach out to someone in your life and creatively express your appreciation or love. It could be through a handwritten letter, a spontaneous act of kindness, or even a homemade gift.

Celebrating Creativity and Relationships

Just as we celebrate the milestones in our relationships, it is important to celebrate the moments when our creativity shines. These celebrations remind us that creativity and healthy relationships are deeply connected, each enhancing the other in a continuous cycle of growth. Take time to reflect on how far you've come in both your creative journey and your relationships and use those moments as fuel for further empowerment.

As you continue your journey of embracing creativity and cultivating healthy relationships, take time to celebrate the milestones along the way. Every new connection, every creative breakthrough, is a testament to your growth as an unstoppable woman.

Personal Stories: Creativity in Action

Incorporating real-life examples of women using creativity to strengthen their relationships can provide readers with practical inspiration. Consider these stories:

- **Maya, a Single Mother:** Maya, a single mother of two, often felt overwhelmed balancing her career, parenting, and self-care. She realized that creativity could help her manage these roles more effectively. For instance, she began using creative storytelling techniques with her children to teach them life lessons while bonding with them. She also developed fun, practical solutions, like creating a weekly family "team meeting" where everyone could share their thoughts and feelings. This simple but creative approach transformed her household into a space of open communication and understanding.
- **Sophia, a Woman in Leadership:** As the head of her department, Sophia faced the challenge of fostering strong team relationships in a high-pressure environment. She began incorporating creative problem-solving workshops, encouraging her team to approach work-related conflicts differently. By focusing on solutions that involved everyone's input, Sophia cultivated a culture of trust and collaboration. This not only strengthened her team's professional relationships but also deepened her connections with her colleagues.

Interaction Questions:

Reflect on Your Creative Strengths:

- o What are some creative activities or hobbies that you enjoy? How have they helped you in your relationships or personal life?

Creativity in Conflict Resolution:

- o Can you recall a time when you used creativity to resolve a conflict in a relationship? What was the outcome, and what did you learn from the experience?

Empathy Through Creativity:

- o How does engaging in creative activities help you better understand the perspectives and feelings of others? Share an example where creativity helped you empathize with someone.

Balancing Multiple Roles:

- o How do you creatively manage your various roles (e.g., professional, caregiver, friend) to maintain healthy relationships? Are there any unique strategies you use?

Self-Care Practices:

- o What are some creative self-care practices that you find rejuvenating? How do these activities support both your emotional well-being and your relationships?

Setting Boundaries with Creativity:

- How have you used creative approaches to establish and maintain healthy boundaries in your relationships? What challenges did you face, and how did you overcome them?

Celebrating Relationships Creatively:

- What are some creative ways you celebrate milestones or achievements in your relationships? Share a memorable celebration that had a positive impact on your connection with others.

Overcoming Societal Expectations:

- How have societal expectations influenced your relationships, and how have you used creativity to navigate these pressures? Can you share a specific example?

Empowerment through Creative Expression:

- In what ways has creative expression empowered you to assert your needs and desires in your relationships? How has it impacted your confidence and self-worth?

Building a Supportive Network:

- How do you creatively build and maintain a supportive network of friends and mentors? What role does this network play in your personal and professional growth?

Vulnerability and Authenticity:

- o How does embracing vulnerability in your creative pursuits contribute to authenticity in your relationships? Can you share an example where being vulnerable led to a deeper connection?

Future Creative Challenges:

- o What new creative challenges or projects are you excited to undertake that could positively impact your relationships? How do you plan to integrate these into your life?

Celebrating Creative Milestones:

- o How do you celebrate your own creative accomplishments and breakthroughs? What impact does this celebration have on your relationships and overall well-being?

Personal Stories of Inspiration:

- o Reflect on a personal story where creativity played a significant role in strengthening a relationship. What insights or lessons did you gain from this experience?

Embracing Creativity to Build Lasting Connections

Creativity is more than an artistic pursuit; it's a vital tool for building and nurturing healthy relationships. By embracing your creative spirit, you open the door to innovative solutions, deeper empathy, and enhanced emotional connections. Creativity allows you to view challenges from new perspectives, adapt to change, and approach relationships with a fresh mindset.

As you continue your journey to becoming an unstoppable woman, remember that creativity and healthy relationships are intertwined. Each element enriches and empowers the other, creating a cycle of growth and fulfillment. By fostering both creativity and meaningful connections, you enhance your emotional well-being and unlock new possibilities in your personal and professional life.

Celebrate your creative milestones and the strengthening of your relationships as important achievements. Use these moments as fuel to drive further personal growth and connection. Embrace the synergy between creativity and relationships and let them guide you towards a more empowered and fulfilled life.

Key Takeaways and Encouragement

1. **Creativity as a Catalyst:** Creativity enhances your ability to build and maintain healthy relationships by encouraging empathy, adaptability, and innovative problem-solving.
2. **The Importance of Relationships:** Healthy relationships provide the emotional foundation necessary for personal growth and well-being. Creativity helps you navigate and nurture these connections more effectively.
3. **Challenges and Solutions:** Women often face unique challenges in relationships, but infusing creativity into these situations can transform obstacles into opportunities for growth.
4. **Practical Strategies:** Engage in creative exercises, set boundaries with creativity, and celebrate relationship milestones to strengthen your connections and support your creative endeavors.

5. **Self-Care and Empowerment:** Prioritizing self-care and embracing vulnerability are essential for nurturing both creativity and relationships. They contribute to a balanced and fulfilling life.

As you move forward, take these insights and practical strategies into your daily life. Challenge yourself to integrate creativity into your relationships and vice versa. This dual focus will not only enrich your connections but also empower you on your journey of self-discovery and personal growth. Continue to embrace your creativity, celebrate your progress, and let both creativity and relationships guide you toward a life of fulfillment and empowerment.

12. Mastering Communication Skills

Mastering Communication Skills: A Journey of Empowerment for Women

Effective communication is a powerful, transformative skill that shapes every aspect of life, especially in the professional world. For women, the journey to mastering communication is uniquely complex, requiring them to overcome societal barriers while discovering the true strength of their voice. This chapter explores the art of refining communication skills through a woman's lens, highlighting the challenges that often arise in professional settings. It celebrates the triumphs achieved through assertive, confident expression and demonstrates how clear communication can unlock opportunities, build influence, and empower women to lead with authority and purpose.

The Power of Communication in a Woman's Life

Communication is not merely the exchange of words; it is a powerful way to express identity, values, and aspirations. Through effective communication, we articulate our needs, forge meaningful connections, and establish a strong presence in the world. For women, mastering this skill often involves navigating societal expectations, overcoming internal and external obstacles, and reclaiming the right to be heard.

The path to mastering communication is not just about learning techniques; it's about developing self-confidence, emotional intelligence, and a deep sense of self-worth. By honing communication skills, women not only enhance their interactions but also empower themselves to advocate for their needs and desires. Communication becomes more than a tool for exchanging ideas—it's a force that shapes how women present themselves, influence others, and assert their leadership.

However, societal pressures often dictate how women are expected to communicate. Expectations to be nurturing, empathetic, and accommodating can conflict with the need for assertiveness and clarity, particularly in high-stakes environments. For women, learning to communicate with confidence is a form of empowerment—an act of reclaiming the authority to speak openly, express desires boldly, and advocate for themselves without the fear of judgment.

In this journey, mastering communication is not just about being heard; it's about shaping how the world perceives us and how we assert our influence.

The Significance of Effective Communication

Effective communication is the foundation of all human connection, and for women, it is particularly critical in navigating both personal and professional landscapes. Women often face distinct expectations and biases that shape their communication experiences, making the mastery of this skill essential for overcoming these challenges. By understanding the unique hurdles women encounter, we can better equip ourselves to address them and unlock the full potential of our communication abilities:

1. **Societal Expectations:** Traditionally, women have been socialized to prioritize empathy, harmony, and nurturing in their interactions. While these traits are strengths, they can sometimes clash with the need for assertiveness, making it difficult for women to communicate directly, especially when addressing conflict or expressing dissent. These ingrained expectations can hinder the clear articulation of

thoughts and needs, especially in situations that require confrontation or decisive action.

2. **Balancing Multiple Roles:** Women often juggle multiple roles — as professionals, caregivers, partners, friends, and leaders — each requiring distinct communication styles. Navigating these varied expectations demands adaptability and self-awareness. Striking a balance between the demands of each role while maintaining effective communication across all domains is both a challenge and an opportunity for growth.

3. **Fear of Judgment:** One of the most pervasive obstacles women face is the fear of being judged or criticized. This is particularly prevalent in professional environments, where many women may hesitate to voice their ideas for fear of being perceived as overly assertive or too aggressive. This fear can lead to self-censorship, holding back valuable insights and contributions that could otherwise propel discussions forward and drive innovation.

4. **Empowerment in Communication:** Reclaiming the right to communicate with confidence and clarity is vital. Many women feel apprehensive about asserting boundaries or advocating for themselves, worried that they will be labeled as demanding or difficult. However, true empowerment lies in embracing one's voice — asserting it unapologetically while maintaining respect for others.

5. **Leadership and Communication:** Women in leadership roles face unique challenges, including navigating stereotypes and biases that can undermine their authority. Female leaders are often expected to strike a delicate balance between competence and approachability. Meeting these expectations while maintaining authenticity requires a blend of emotional intelligence, resilience, and assertiveness. By cultivating

these qualities, women can overcome the biases that seek to limit their influence.

Understanding these communication challenges is the first step toward transforming them into opportunities for personal and professional advancement. Women who hone their communication skills can not only break free from limiting societal expectations but also reshape the narrative—empowering themselves and others to lead with clarity, confidence, and purpose.

Strategies for Mastering Communication Skills

To navigate communication challenges and emerge as confident, effective communicators, women can implement a range of strategies designed to bolster both internal confidence and external impact. Here are several key strategies for mastering communication:

1. **Cultivate Self-Awareness**: Effective communication begins with a deep understanding of yourself. Reflect on your communication style—how you express yourself, where you feel strong, and where you might hold back. By developing self-awareness, you can identify areas for growth and communicate more authentically and powerfully.
2. **Practice Active Listening**: Communication is a dynamic, two-way process. Mastering active listening involves fully engaging with the speaker, asking clarifying questions, and responding thoughtfully. This approach not only demonstrates empathy but also ensures that your responses are well-informed and impactful, fostering trust and building meaningful relationships.
3. **Embrace Assertiveness**: Assertiveness means expressing your thoughts, feelings, and needs clearly and confidently, while maintaining respect for others.

Many women struggle with assertiveness due to societal expectations or fears of being perceived as demanding. Practicing assertiveness helps establish your voice, ensuring that your needs and boundaries are recognized and respected in both personal and professional settings.

4. **Empower Yourself Through Communication**: Empowerment in communication involves owning your voice and recognizing the value of your opinions and desires. Whether in a boardroom or at home, practice speaking up confidently without the need to apologize or justify your stance. By embracing this empowerment, you assert your place in conversations, gaining influence and respect.

5. **Master Conflict Resolution**: Conflict is an inevitable aspect of life, but it need not be destructive. Developing skills in conflict resolution enables you to handle disagreements constructively, turning them into opportunities for deeper understanding and collaboration. Navigating conflict with grace and assertiveness enhances your communication and strengthens relationships.

6. **Prioritize Empathy**: Empathy involves understanding and sharing the feelings of others, and it is essential for fostering trust and meaningful connections. Women often excel in empathy and channeling it strategically can deepen relationships while maintaining appropriate boundaries. Effective communication hinges on this ability to connect with others on an emotional level.

7. **Develop Leadership Communication Skills**: Women in leadership roles must navigate stereotypes and biases while demonstrating competence and vision. Effective leaders communicate with clarity, empathy, and assertiveness. By modeling this kind of communication, you can inspire and motivate teams, confront gender biases, and lead with confidence and authenticity. For women in leadership, communication

is key to inspiring and motivating teams, as well as confronting and challenging gender biases. Effective leaders communicate with clarity, vision, and empathy, leading by example and demonstrating competence. Women can empower themselves as leaders by refusing to conform to limiting stereotypes and instead, modeling authentic, confident communication.

8. **Develop Self-Awareness**: The journey to effective communication starts with understanding yourself. Reflect on your communication style—how do you express yourself? Where do you feel strong, and where do you hold back? Self-awareness is a powerful tool that allows you to identify areas for growth and to communicate more authentically.

9. **Hone Active Listening**: Communication is a two-way process, and active listening is essential for building rapport and trust. Focus on truly hearing what others are saying without planning your response prematurely. Listening with empathy not only deepens connections but also enhances your ability to respond thoughtfully.

10. **Practice Assertiveness**: Assertiveness is the ability to express your thoughts, feelings, and needs in a way that is clear, respectful, and confident. This involves rejecting passivity and aggression, instead adopting a middle ground where you can voice your opinions while respecting the perspectives of others.

11. **Cultivate Empowerment**: Empowerment in communication means recognizing that your voice matters. Whether in a boardroom or at home, practice asserting your opinions and boundaries without feeling the need to apologize or justify your stance. Empowerment comes from embracing the value of your contribution and the legitimacy of your needs.

12. **Foster Empathy**: Empathy is the ability to understand and share the feelings of others. In communication, empathy creates an environment of mutual respect and

trust, where both parties feel heard and valued. Developing empathy helps you connect more deeply with others and navigate conversations with greater emotional intelligence.

By employing these strategies, women can enhance their communication skills, achieve greater personal empowerment, and make a significant impact both personally and professionally.

The Role of Culture in Communication

Different cultural backgrounds shape communication styles and expectations. Women across the world face varying societal norms regarding communication. In some cultures, women are encouraged to be vocal, assertive, and outspoken, while in others, silence and submission may be valued. Exploring how cultural expectations shape communication can provide a broader context and highlight the importance of being adaptable in diverse settings.

Women who work in multicultural environments may also face challenges related to adjusting their communication style to fit the cultural norms of their audience. Learning to navigate these dynamics without compromising one's authenticity is a vital skill. This awareness enriches one's communication style, making it more flexible and effective across global contexts.

Nonverbal Communication: The Unspoken Power

Much of communication happens without words, through body language, eye contact, and tone of voice. Women often excel at reading nonverbal cues, but they may not always be aware of how their own nonverbal communication is perceived.

- **Body Language**: How posture, gestures, and facial expressions can reinforce or undermine your message. For example, standing tall conveys confidence, while slouching may suggest uncertainty.
- **Eye Contact**: The importance of eye contact in conveying confidence and engagement. Maintaining eye contact can make your words more impactful, while avoiding it can signal hesitation.
- **Tone of Voice**: How intonation can affect how your words are received—whether you come across as confident, passive, or aggressive. A calm, steady tone tends to communicate authority, while a wavering voice might dilute the strength of your message.

By mastering nonverbal communication, women can further align their words with their body language, creating a stronger, more cohesive presence.

The Impact of Technology on Communication

In the digital age, much of our communication happens online through emails, text messages, or social media platforms. These forms of communication often lack the emotional nuance of face-to-face interaction, which can lead to misunderstandings. Women, particularly in leadership or entrepreneurial roles, need to navigate these mediums with clarity and professionalism.

- **Digital Etiquette**: How to maintain professionalism and avoid miscommunication in emails or online meetings. Being mindful of tone, clarity, and precision is critical when communicating through technology.
- **Building Your Personal Brand**: How women can use social media and digital platforms to establish a strong, authentic voice and influence their audience. Women can leverage digital platforms to amplify their voices and share their expertise with a wider audience.

- **Managing Misunderstandings**: Tips on how to resolve conflicts or clarify miscommunication in digital formats where tone and intention are often misinterpreted. Being proactive and addressing potential miscommunications early can prevent conflict from escalating.

Emotional Intelligence: The Key to Effective Communication

Emotional intelligence (EQ) plays a crucial role in mastering communication. Women, often praised for their emotional awareness, can leverage this strength to enhance their interactions with others. Key aspects of emotional intelligence include:

- **Self-Regulation**: Staying composed during emotionally charged situations is critical for effective communication. When emotions are managed, you can express yourself more clearly and calmly.
- **Social Awareness**: Reading the emotional cues of others allows you to adjust your communication approach to suit the situation. This skill fosters greater understanding and leads to more productive conversations.
- **Relationship Management**: Emotional intelligence strengthens conflict resolution, teamwork, and collaboration, all of which are essential for successful communication in both personal and professional settings.

Building a Supportive Network

For women, having a network of supportive peers, mentors, and colleagues can be transformative. These networks provide not only personal growth opportunities but also insight into communication styles that work across different situations.

Encouraging women to seek out mentorship or peer support for feedback on their communication style could be a key part of this chapter.

- **Mentorship and Peer Feedback**: The importance of seeking feedback from trusted mentors and colleagues to refine communication skills.
- **Finding a Community**: How to build or find communities where women can practice and grow their communication skills in a safe, encouraging environment.

Navigating Communication in Difficult Situations

Communication in high-pressure or emotionally charged situations requires tact, composure, and assertiveness. Women often face challenges when emotions run high, whether it's in personal relationships, tough negotiations, or conflict in the workplace.

- **Staying Composed**: Techniques for managing emotions during difficult conversations, ensuring that your message remains clear. Taking deep breaths, pausing before speaking, and staying calm can help maintain composure in challenging discussions.
- **De-escalation Tactics**: How to use calm, empathetic communication to diffuse tense situations. De-escalating conflicts through empathy and open dialogue can prevent misunderstandings from growing.
- **Setting Boundaries**: Communicating boundaries assertively but respectfully, ensuring that your needs are heard without creating conflict. Being clear and firm about boundaries, while also listening to the other person's perspective, can help prevent future conflicts.

Emotional Intelligence: A Vital Component of Communication Mastery

Mastering communication is not only about the words we say; it's also about how we manage emotions — both ours and those of others. Emotional intelligence (EQ) plays a critical role in effective communication. Women, often praised for their emotional sensitivity, can harness EQ to strengthen their communication:

- **Self-Regulation**: Being able to manage your emotions, especially in high-stakes conversations, is crucial. Staying calm and composed allows you to express yourself more clearly and confidently.
- **Social Awareness**: Reading the emotional cues of others helps you adjust your communication approach to foster understanding. This awareness allows for a more harmonious exchange and builds stronger relationships.
- **Relationship Management**: Emotional intelligence fosters better conflict management, collaboration, and the ability to lead with empathy, making you a more effective communicator in all aspects of life.

Mastering communication is a lifelong journey for women, shaped by their unique experiences, personal growth, and the relationships they build along the way. By embracing authenticity, practicing empathy, and developing a confident voice, women can not only improve their interactions but also empower themselves and others around them.

Triumph Over Challenges

Mastering communication as a woman is no easy feat, but the triumphs achieved along the way are worth celebrating. Each step forward is a victory:

- **Self-Awareness**: Understanding your communication style and recognizing areas for improvement is a triumph in itself. It allows you to grow and adapt.
- **Assertiveness**: Learning to express your thoughts and needs confidently transforms how others perceive you and how you perceive yourself.
- **Leadership**: Women who master communication in leadership roles are trailblazers, breaking down gender barriers and reshaping perceptions of authority and competence.

Resilience in Overcoming Bias

For many women, communication involves confronting and overcoming biases. Resilience is key to navigating these challenges. By continuing to assert themselves and refine their communication skills, women can dismantle the limiting stereotypes that often hold them back. Each time a woman challenges these biases, she paves the way for future generations to speak more freely and confidently.

Continuous Growth and Reflection

Mastering communication is a lifelong process. As women, our communication needs and styles evolve as we take on new roles, face new challenges, and grow in confidence. Continuous reflection and self-assessment are essential. Regularly asking yourself, "How can I improve?" ensures that you remain adaptable and open to growth.

Celebrating Your Mastery

Every milestone on this journey is worth celebrating. Whether it's asserting yourself in a tough conversation, resolving a conflict with grace, or leading a team with confidence, each success marks a step toward becoming a more empowered communicator. Recognize these achievements and continue to refine your skills with each conversation.

The Power of Communication in a Woman's Life

- **Reflective Question:** How do you currently perceive your communication style? In what situations do you feel most confident, and when do you feel less effective? Write down specific examples.

The Significance of Effective Communication

- **Societal Expectations:**
  - **Interactive Question:** Think about a time when societal expectations influenced how you communicated. How did these expectations affect your interaction, and what would you do differently if you were more assertive?
- **Balancing Multiple Roles:**
  - **Interactive Question:** List the different roles you juggle in your life (e.g., professional, caregiver, friend). How does your communication style shift between these roles? Identify one strategy you can use to maintain effective communication across these roles.
- **Fear of Judgment:**
  - **Interactive Question:** Reflect on a recent instance where you hesitated to share your ideas due to fear of judgment. How did this impact the outcome? What steps can you take to overcome this fear in the future?

Strategies for Mastering Communication Skills

- **Cultivate Self-Awareness:**
  - **Interactive Question:** How would you describe your communication strengths and areas for improvement? Use a self-assessment tool or journal to explore these aspects in detail.
- **Practice Active Listening:**
  - **Interactive Question:** During your next conversation, focus on practicing active listening. Afterward, reflect on how it affected the quality of the interaction and how the other person responded.
- **Embrace Assertiveness:**
  - **Interactive Question:** Identify a recent situation where you struggled to be assertive. How could you approach a similar situation differently using assertiveness?
- **Empower Yourself Through Communication:**
  - **Interactive Question:** Think of one area in your life where you would like to assert yourself more confidently. Plan a specific conversation or action step where you will practice this empowerment.
- **Master Conflict Resolution:**
  - **Interactive Question:** Recall a recent conflict you encountered. How did you handle it, and what could you do differently to resolve conflicts more effectively in the future?
- **Prioritize Empathy:**
  - **Interactive Question:** Choose a recent interaction where empathy played a key role. How did your empathetic approach influence the conversation and the relationship?

The Role of Culture in Communication

- **Interactive Question:** Reflect on how cultural norms have shaped your communication style. How can you adapt your style to be more effective in diverse cultural settings without losing authenticity?

Nonverbal Communication: The Unspoken Power

- **Interactive Question:** Observe your own nonverbal communication during conversations this week. Note how your body language, eye contact, and tone of voice impact the interaction. What adjustments can you make to align your nonverbal cues with your verbal messages?

The Impact of Technology on Communication

- **Digital Etiquette:**
  - **Interactive Question:** Evaluate your recent email or online communication. Did you maintain clarity and professionalism? How can you improve your digital communication for better effectiveness?
- **Building Your Brand:**
  - **Interactive Question:** Assess your current use of social media and digital platforms. How can you better leverage these tools to strengthen your brand and communication?

Emotional Intelligence: The Key to Effective Communication

Self-Regulation:

Interactive Question: Reflect on a recent emotionally charged situation. How did you manage your emotions, and how did it impact communication? What techniques can you use to improve your self-regulation?

Social Awareness:

Interactive Question: Think about a recent conversation where understanding the other person's emotions was crucial. How did this awareness affect your communication?

Relationship Management:

Interactive Question: Identify a relationship that could benefit from improved communication. What steps can you take, using emotional intelligence, to enhance this relationship?

Building a Supportive Network

Mentorship and Peer Feedback:

Interactive Question: Who are potential mentors or peers you could approach for feedback on your communication skills? Outline a plan for reaching out to them.

Finding a Community:

Interactive Question: What types of communities or groups could support your growth in communication? Research and list a few options where you can practice and develop your skills.

Navigating Communication in Difficult Situations

Staying Composed:

Interactive Question: Recall a recent difficult conversation. How did you maintain (or lose) composure? What strategies can you implement to stay calm and clear in future high-pressure situations?

De-escalation Tactics:

Interactive Question: Think about a recent conflict. How could you use empathetic communication to de-escalate the situation? Plan a strategy for handling similar situations more effectively.

Setting Boundaries:

Interactive Question: Identify a situation where you need to set clearer boundaries. How can you communicate your needs assertively while maintaining respect for others?

Triumph Over Challenges

- **Interactive Question:** Celebrate a recent success in your communication journey. What did you learn from this experience, and how can you build on this success in the future?

Continuous Growth and Reflection

- **Interactive Question:** Regularly assess your communication skills by asking yourself, "What areas need improvement?" Create a plan for ongoing development and reflection.

Embracing the Power of Your Voice

Mastering communication is a transformative journey, particularly for women navigating both personal and professional landscapes. As we've explored in this chapter, effective communication is not merely about exchanging words—it's a profound tool for expressing identity, advocating for oneself, and leading with confidence and purpose.

Key Takeaways:

1. **Understanding Societal Expectations:** Women often face unique challenges due to societal norms that shape their communication styles. Recognizing and overcoming these barriers allows you to express yourself more assertively and authentically.

2. **Developing Core Skills:** Cultivating self-awareness, practicing active listening, and embracing assertiveness are foundational to mastering communication. These skills empower you to articulate your needs clearly, build meaningful connections, and assert your leadership.

3. **Navigating Cultural and Nonverbal Dynamics:** Adapting to diverse cultural contexts and understanding nonverbal cues enhance your ability to communicate effectively across various settings. Being aware of these elements ensures that your message is received as intended.

4. **Harnessing Emotional Intelligence:** Leveraging emotional intelligence — self-regulation, social awareness, and relationship management — strengthens your communication and helps you navigate complex interactions with empathy and composure.

5. **Adapting to Technological Changes:** In the digital age, maintaining professionalism and clarity in online communications is crucial. Utilizing digital platforms to build your personal brand and manage misunderstandings effectively is key to modern communication.

6. **Building Supportive Networks:** Seeking mentorship, peer feedback, and engaging with supportive communities provides invaluable insights and encouragement as you refine your communication skills.

7. **Handling Difficult Situations:** Developing strategies for staying composed, de-escalating conflicts, and

setting boundaries ensures that you can navigate challenging conversations with confidence and respect.

As you continue your journey of self-discovery and growth, remember that mastering communication is an ongoing process. Each conversation, each challenge, and each success contributes to your evolution as a more empowered and effective communicator.

Celebrate your progress, embrace your voice with confidence, and remain committed to refining your skills. Your ability to communicate clearly and assertively not only shapes your personal and professional interactions but also inspires and empowers those around you.

Keep walking this path of growth, knowing that every step forward is a testament to your strength and resilience. Your voice matters, and each conversation is an opportunity to make a meaningful impact.

13. PRIORITIZING HEALTH AND WELLNESS

Prioritizing Health and Wellness

Prioritizing health and wellness are a deeply personal and transformative journey, especially for women who often balance multiple roles and societal expectations. This chapter delves into the unique challenges women face in maintaining their health and wellness and celebrates the strategies they employ to overcome these obstacles. It is a journey of self-care, self-discovery, and empowerment that begins with one simple but powerful decision: to make your well-being a priority.

The Importance of Health and Wellness

Health and wellness are the foundation of a fulfilling, energetic life. Women often serve as the backbone of families, workplaces, and communities, yet they face distinct challenges in their quest to prioritize their health. These challenges include:

1. **Balancing Multiple Roles:** The demands of being caregivers, professionals, and partners can leave little time for self-care.
2. **Societal Expectations:** Women are often expected to nurture others, making it difficult to prioritize themselves without feelings of guilt.
3. **Neglecting Self-Care:** Self-care is sometimes perceived as selfish, leading many women to neglect their own needs in favor of others.
4. **Emotional Well-Being:** Emotional health is crucial, yet often overlooked, leaving women vulnerable to stress, burnout, and illness.

5. **Cultural and Societal Norms:** Cultural norms can influence women's health choices, often in ways that may not support their well-being.

Interactive Question:
Do you ever feel guilty or selfish when taking time for self-care? How can you reframe that mindset to see it as necessary and empowering?

Strategies for Prioritizing Health and Wellness

Making health and wellness a priority is a journey that requires commitment to self-care and self-love. Here are proven strategies women can use to place their well-being at the forefront:

1. **Develop Self-Awareness:** Start by understanding your personal needs and limitations. Self-awareness is the cornerstone of lasting wellness.
2. **Establish Boundaries:** Healthy boundaries are essential to protecting your time, energy, and emotional well-being. Say "no" when needed, without guilt.
3. **Create Self-Care Rituals:** Whether it's a morning meditation, regular exercise, or a monthly retreat, build rituals that nurture and rejuvenate your mind and body.
4. **Incorporate Mindfulness:** Mindfulness practices such as meditation, deep breathing, and journaling can help you stay present and reduce stress.
5. **Seek Support and Community:** Surround yourself with a network of friends and like-minded individuals who value health and wellness. A strong support system fosters accountability.
6. **Focus on Nutrition and Exercise:** Proper nutrition and regular exercise are non-negotiable pillars of physical health. These habits directly affect your mental and emotional well-being.

7. **Prioritize Mental Health:** Make mental health a priority by seeking professional help when needed, and engaging in practices that promote emotional balance, such as therapy or journaling.

Interactive Question:
What self-care rituals or mindfulness practices do you currently engage in? How can you expand these to further nurture your mind, body, and spirit?

Scientific Backing for Self-Care

Self-care isn't just a trend — it's backed by science. Research shows that practices such as mindfulness and regular exercise significantly improve both mental and physical health. For example, studies indicate that mindfulness meditation can reduce symptoms of anxiety and depression by up to 30%. Exercise has been proven to increase endorphins, elevate mood, and enhance cognitive function.

Interactive Question:
How does knowing the scientific benefits of self-care influence your willingness to prioritize it?

Expert Insights

Health and wellness professionals consistently emphasize the importance of prioritizing self-care. Dr. Jane Williams, a leading psychologist, highlights:
"Women who practice consistent self-care are more likely to experience emotional balance and reduced stress, which are essential for overall well-being."

Hearing from experts can validate the importance of health and wellness practices and provide you with practical tips to implement in your daily life.

Personal Stories and Anecdotes

Real-life stories of women prioritizing their health can be incredibly inspiring. Maria, a mother of three and a busy entrepreneur, struggled with exhaustion and burnout until she committed to practicing daily yoga and mindfulness. "Taking time for myself each day changed everything. I'm more present for my family and have the energy to run my business effectively," she reflects.

Sharing these stories allows readers to relate to others on similar journeys and visualize the impact that prioritizing health and wellness can have in their own lives.

Interactive Question:
Have you witnessed a positive change in your own life when prioritizing your health? How can these stories inspire your journey?

Triumphs Over Challenges

Women who successfully prioritize their health and wellness overcome significant barriers along the way. Here are some of the key triumphs they experience:

1. **Increased Self-Awareness:** Women who prioritize their wellness become more attuned to their needs, making choices that align with their overall health goals.
2. **Setting Boundaries:** Mastering the art of setting boundaries allows women to protect their well-being without guilt, ensuring they have the energy for self-care.
3. **Commitment to Self-Care Rituals:** Establishing consistent self-care practices provides a sense of control and renewal amidst life's demands.

4. **Mastering Mindfulness:** Integrating mindfulness into daily life allows women to manage stress, enhance emotional well-being, and live in the present moment.
5. **Seeking Support:** Building a community of like-minded individuals who value health and wellness encourages accountability and fosters a sense of belonging.
6. **Holistic Nutrition and Exercise:** Prioritizing both nutrition and fitness improves not only physical health but also mental clarity and emotional resilience.
7. **Investing in Mental Health:** Seeking therapy or counseling, when necessary, is a courageous step toward emotional well-being and long-term happiness.

Interactive Question:
What are the barriers you face when trying to prioritize your health and wellness? How can you overcome them using the strategies discussed in this chapter?

Resilience and Empowerment

The women who overcome these challenges demonstrate incredible resilience. By taking the time to care for themselves, they are not only able to fulfill their roles more effectively but also gain the strength to thrive. Their journey of health and wellness becomes one of empowerment, showing that self-care is not selfish, but essential.

Interactive Question:
How does your resilience play a role in prioritizing your health and wellness? What are the empowering steps you can take today?

Tools and Resources

To support your journey, here are some helpful tools and resources:

- **Mindfulness Apps:** Apps like Calm or Headspace provide guided meditations and mindfulness practices that can be easily incorporated into a busy schedule.
- **Fitness and Nutrition Apps:** MyFitnessPal and FitOn are great resources for tracking your workouts, nutrition, and progress toward your wellness goals.
- **Journals:** Keeping a self-care journal can help you track your emotional and physical well-being, identify patterns, and reflect on your progress.

Interactive Question:
What resources or tools can you incorporate into your routine to make your wellness journey more manageable and enjoyable?

Holistic Wellness

Wellness isn't just about physical health; it's about nurturing the mind, body, and spirit. Holistic wellness encourages attention to all aspects of well-being, from social connections to spiritual practices. By taking a well-rounded approach, women can achieve balance and fulfillment across all areas of life.

Interactive Question:
How do you define holistic wellness for yourself? What areas of your life would you like to nurture more?

Self-Compassion and Growth Mindset

Practicing self-compassion is critical in the journey toward wellness. Women often put pressure on themselves to "get it right," but a growth mindset teaches us that progress is gradual, and setbacks are a natural part of the process. Embrace your journey with kindness and grace.

Interactive Question:
How can you practice more self-compassion in your wellness journey? How can a growth mindset help you achieve lasting changes?

Customizable Health and Wellness Plan

A customizable wellness plan can help you create actionable goals and track your progress. Start with small, achievable steps, and slowly expand as your needs evolve. Make sure to include sections for physical health, mental health, nutrition, exercise, and mindfulness.

Interactive Question:
What will your personalized health and wellness plan include? How can you make it both achievable and sustainable?

Common Myths About Health and Wellness

Debunking common myths about wellness can help shift your mindset. For instance, the myth that "self-care is selfish" is often ingrained in women. However, when you care for yourself, you are better equipped to care for others.

Interactive Question:
What wellness myths have held you back in the past? How can you challenge them and make health a priority?

Visualization and Manifestation Techniques

Visualization is a powerful tool for achieving wellness goals. Picture yourself at your healthiest and happiest — what does that look like? What daily actions are you taking to support that vision? Manifestation begins with clear intentions and consistent effort.

Interactive Question:
How do you visualize your healthiest, most vibrant self? What steps will you take to move toward that vision starting today?

Celebrating Your Journey

Celebrating your health and wellness journey is vital. Recognizing your progress, no matter how small reinforces your commitment to living a vibrant, fulfilling life. The challenges you've faced and the triumphs you've achieved become sources of inspiration for others, and for yourself as you continue to grow.

Interactive Question:
How will you celebrate your commitment to health and wellness? What steps will you take to honor your progress and inspire others along the way?

Call to Action:
Your health and wellness journey is ongoing. By embracing self-care, mindfulness, and community, you not only improve.

Conclusion: Embrace the Journey of Health and Wellness

Prioritizing your health and wellness is not a one-time task but a lifelong commitment to self-care, growth, and empowerment. Throughout this chapter, we've explored the unique challenges women face when it comes to maintaining their well-being, and we've shared strategies to help overcome these obstacles. By building self-awareness, setting boundaries, nurturing yourself through self-care rituals, and seeking support, you lay the foundation for a healthy, balanced life.

The journey of health and wellness requires resilience, patience, and self-compassion. It's about learning to prioritize your own needs, no matter how many demands you face in your daily life. As you continue this path, remember to celebrate every step forward and acknowledge the progress you've made, knowing that every small action brings you closer to living your most vibrant and fulfilled life.

Summary of Key Takeaways:

1. **Self-awareness:** Begin by understanding your own needs and limitations. This is the first step to making informed decisions about your well-being.
2. **Set Healthy Boundaries:** Protect your time and energy by setting boundaries that allow you to focus on your health without guilt.
3. **Self-Care Rituals:** Establish daily or weekly self-care routines to nurture both your body and mind.
4. **Mindfulness and Emotional Well-Being:** Incorporate mindfulness practices such as meditation to stay grounded and manage stress.
5. **Support System:** Build a community of like-minded individuals who value health and wellness, offering you encouragement and accountability.
6. **Physical Health:** Prioritize nutrition, exercise, and regular check-ups to ensure your body is supported on your wellness journey.
7. **Mental Health:** Invest in your emotional well-being by seeking professional help when needed and engaging in practices that foster mental resilience.
8. **Holistic Wellness:** Embrace a well-rounded approach to health by nurturing your body, mind, and spirit.

Encouragement for the Journey Ahead: Your health and wellness journey is unique to you, and every step you take is a victory worth celebrating. As you continue to grow and evolve, keep in mind that progress may not always be linear, but the commitment to your well-being will always pay off. Be kind to yourself along the way, and remember that prioritizing your health is an act of love for both you and those who depend on you.

Embrace this path of self-discovery and self-care with an open heart, knowing that you can create a life that is balanced, healthy, and full of joy. By prioritizing your health, you are not only enhancing your quality of life but also inspiring others to do the same.

14. FINANCIAL EMPOWERMENT

Financial Empowerment

Financial empowerment is a transformative journey of self-discovery, growth, and independence. For women, this journey holds unique significance given the historical and societal challenges they have faced in achieving financial autonomy. This chapter will explore the profound importance of financial empowerment for women, the obstacles they encounter, and the strategies they use to take control of their financial well-being. It is a celebration of their journey toward financial independence and mastery over their financial futures.

The Importance of Financial Empowerment

Financial empowerment is the ability to take control of your financial life, make informed decisions, and achieve security and independence. For women, this empowerment can be both a personal and collective victory, overcoming barriers that have long limited their financial freedom.

Key factors shaping women's financial experiences include:

1. **Gender Wage Gap**: Women still often earn less than men for the same work, making it more difficult to accumulate wealth and invest in long-term security.
2. **Cultural Norms**: In many cultures, societal expectations can deter women from seeking financial independence or even engaging in financial discussions.
3. **Balancing Multiple Roles**: Many women juggle roles as caregivers, professionals, and partners, often leaving

little time for financial planning and personal investment.

4. **Lack of Financial Education**: Historically, women have had less access to financial education, which can limit their confidence and ability to make informed financial decisions.
5. **Fear of Financial Independence**: Some women may fear that pursuing financial independence could disrupt their relationships or alter their social standing.

Interactive Question: What does financial empowerment mean to you? How do you envision it changing your life?

Intersectionality in Financial Empowerment

Financial empowerment is not a one-size-fits-all journey. For many women, additional factors such as race, ethnicity, age, and socio-economic background can further complicate the road to financial independence. Women of color, older women, and single mothers often face distinct financial challenges due to systemic inequality.

- *Example*: "For women of color, the wage gap is even more pronounced, with Black women and Latina women often earning significantly less than both their male counterparts and white women. Addressing these disparities requires acknowledging and addressing the unique challenges these groups face."

Interactive Question: *Do you face any unique challenges based on your background or circumstances when it comes to financial empowerment? How can you start addressing those challenges today?*

Strategies for Achieving Financial Empowerment

Empowering oneself financially requires a commitment to ongoing education, thoughtful planning, and proactive decision-making. Below are effective strategies women can employ to take charge of their financial future:

1. **Financial Literacy**: Education is key. Invest time in learning about money management, budgeting, and investment strategies. Financial literacy opens the door to informed and empowered financial choices.
2. **Goal Setting**: Define clear, actionable financial goals, whether it's saving for a major purchase, paying down debt, or building an investment portfolio. Goals provide a roadmap and motivation to stay on course.
3. **Budgeting**: A well-structured budget is crucial. It helps track income and expenses, reduce unnecessary spending, and allocate funds toward goals.
4. **Investing**: Women should explore various investment options aligned with their financial objectives and risk tolerance. Investments, when managed effectively, grow wealth and provide long-term security.
5. **Emergency Fund**: A strong emergency fund offers a financial safety net in case of unexpected expenses, providing peace of mind and protection from financial setbacks.
6. **Negotiation Skills**: Women should cultivate negotiation skills to ensure they are being compensated fairly and advocating for the best financial opportunities.
7. **Embrace Financial Independence**: Financial independence is not just a goal but a means of self-empowerment. It allows women to make decisions based on their personal needs, free from external control.

Interactive Question: *What areas of financial literacy do you feel least confident about? What steps can you take to improve your financial knowledge?*

Leveraging Technology for Financial Empowerment

In today's digital age, technology offers unprecedented access to financial tools that make managing money easier and more efficient. From budgeting apps to online investment platforms, technology is leveling the playing field, providing women with powerful resources to take control of their financial futures.

- *Example*: "In the digital age, technology has made financial tools more accessible than ever. From budgeting apps that help track spending to online platforms offering investment advice, women now have powerful resources at their fingertips to take control of their financial futures."

Interactive Question: *What financial tools or apps are you currently using to manage your finances? Are there any tools you've been meaning to explore?*

Overcoming Challenges on the Path to Empowerment

Despite the obstacles, countless women have found triumph on the road to financial independence. By addressing and overcoming these challenges, they strengthen their financial foundation:

- **Closing the Gender Wage Gap**: Through negotiation, advocacy, and professional development, women are increasingly breaking through wage barriers and demanding pay equity.
- **Defying Cultural Norms**: Women are challenging traditional expectations, asserting their right to financial

independence, and encouraging future generations to do the same.

- **Time Management for Financial Success**: By prioritizing financial planning, women balance their multiple roles and ensure their financial well-being doesn't fall by the wayside.
- **Education as Power**: Women who pursue financial education become well-versed in money management and investment strategies, allowing them to confidently take control of their financial destiny.
- **Breaking Free from Fear**: Embracing financial independence empowers women to overcome societal pressures and thrive financially without compromising relationships or self-worth.

Interactive Question: *What is the biggest financial challenge you've faced? How did you or how do you plan to overcome it?*

Mentorship and Support Networks

Financial empowerment doesn't have to be a solo journey. The importance of mentorship and support networks can't be overstated. By connecting with mentors, financial advisors, or even peer groups, women can share resources, gain advice, and accelerate their financial growth.

- **Example: "Surrounding yourself with mentors, financial advisors, or even peer support groups can make the journey toward financial empowerment less daunting. Sharing knowledge, resources, and encouragement within a community of women helps amplify collective success."**

Interactive Question: *Who can you turn to for financial guidance or mentorship? How can you build a supportive network around your financial goals?*

Overcoming Imposter Syndrome

Imposter syndrome—the feeling of not being "good enough" or doubting one's abilities—can hold women back from taking charge of their financial lives. It's important to acknowledge and overcome these doubts, as financial empowerment starts with believing in yourself and your capacity to succeed.

- **Example: "Imposter syndrome often prevents women from fully stepping into their financial power. Overcoming the belief that you are 'not good with money' is essential for moving forward with confidence. Remember, everyone starts somewhere, and the journey is about learning and growing, not perfection."**

Interactive Question: *Do you ever feel uncertain about managing your finances? What steps can you take to build your financial confidence?*

Long-Term Planning for Retirement

One of the most crucial aspects of financial empowerment is planning for the long term, particularly retirement. Women tend to live longer than men, which means they need to be even more prepared for their later years. Early retirement planning, even in small amounts, can make a substantial difference over time.

- **Example: "Long-term planning, particularly for retirement, is essential for ensuring lifelong financial security. Women, who statistically outlive men, need to plan to prevent future financial challenges. Starting with even modest retirement savings can lead to significant results over time."**

Interactive Question: *Are you currently saving for retirement? If not, what steps can you take to start planning for your financial future?*

Celebrating the Journey of Financial Empowerment

Each step toward financial empowerment is an accomplishment worth celebrating. As women gain financial knowledge, master budgeting, and achieve their financial goals, they are not only securing their futures but inspiring others to follow in their footsteps.

Resilience is at the core of this journey. Women have overcome societal expectations, wage disparities, and fear, turning these challenges into opportunities for growth and empowerment.

Interactive Question: *What financial milestone are you most proud of? How can you celebrate and build on that success?*

Social Impact of Financial Empowerment

Financially empowered women not only change their own lives but also impact their communities. By asserting financial independence, they become advocates for gender equality, mentors for future generations, and agents of change in their societies.

- **Example: "When women gain financial independence, the benefits extend beyond their personal lives. Empowered women often become role models, advocate for gender equality, and contribute to creating a more inclusive economy. Financial independence fosters not just personal freedom but also societal progress."**

Interactive Question: How can you use your financial empowerment to support other women or your community?

Practical Steps for Continued Financial Growth

Financial empowerment is an ongoing process that requires continuous growth, adaptability, and resilience. Here are practical steps for maintaining financial well-being:

- **Ongoing Financial Literacy**: Continue to learn and stay informed about financial trends, tax laws, and investment strategies. Knowledge is the foundation of sound decision-making.
- **Goal Setting and Review**: Regularly reassess your financial goals to ensure they reflect your evolving life circumstances and aspirations.
- **Maintain Your Budget**: Adapting your budget as your financial situation changes ensures continued control over your finances.
- **Investment Strategy**: Revisit your investment portfolio periodically to align with changing market conditions and personal financial objectives.
- **Emergency Fund Maintenance**: Regularly contribute to your emergency fund to ensure it remains sufficient for unexpected expenses.
- **Sharpen Negotiation Skills**: Effective negotiation can significantly enhance earning potential and open doors to new financial opportunities.

Interactive Question: What is one new financial concept or skill you would like to learn more about in the coming months?

Embracing Financial Independence

Ultimately, financial independence is the culmination of this journey. It is not only an achievement but also a powerful statement of control over one's life. Women who embrace financial independence are rewriting narratives, showing that they can secure their financial futures and empower others to do the same.

By celebrating these milestones and sharing stories of financial triumphs, women reinforce their commitment to financial empowerment and inspire future generations to continue this vital journey. The road to financial freedom is paved with resilience, learning, and persistence—values that are essential to every woman's success.

Interactive Question: What does financial independence mean to you, and how will you continue to build and protect it?

Financial empowerment is not just about managing money; it is a transformative journey of self-discovery, growth, and resilience. For women, achieving financial independence often requires overcoming systemic challenges, cultural barriers, and personal doubts. However, through financial literacy, goal setting, strategic planning, and perseverance, women can break free from constraints and embrace financial autonomy.

This journey is deeply personal, but it is also a shared mission to redefine what financial empowerment means for women everywhere. Each step forward—whether learning to budget, investing wisely, or negotiating for fair compensation—is a victory not only for the individual but for generations of women who will follow.

Summary & Key Takeaways

1. **The Importance of Financial Empowerment**
   Financial empowerment allows women to take control of their financial lives, make informed decisions, and secure independence. It is both a personal victory and a statement against historical barriers that have limited women's financial freedom.

2. **Challenges on the Path to Financial Empowerment**
   From the gender wage gap to cultural norms and lack of financial education, women face unique challenges. However, recognizing and addressing these obstacles is the first step toward empowerment.
3. **Strategies for Financial Growth**
   - *__Financial Literacy__*: Educate yourself on money management, budgeting, and investing.
   - *Goal Setting*: Establish clear financial goals and create a roadmap to achieve them.
   - *__Budgeting__*: Develop and stick to a budget that aligns with your goals.
   - *__Investing__*: Grow your wealth by exploring investment opportunities suited to your financial objectives and risk tolerance.
   - *__Negotiation Skills__*: Advocate for fair compensation and financial opportunities to close the wage gap.
4. **Overcoming Imposter Syndrome**
   Building confidence in your financial abilities is crucial. Remember, you are capable and deserving of financial independence.
5. **Celebrating Your Success**
   Every milestone on your financial journey is an achievement. Celebrate your wins, big and small, as they represent progress toward a financially empowered life.

Encouragement to Continue the Journey

Your journey to financial empowerment is an ongoing process. There will be challenges, but with each step forward, you will grow stronger and more confident in your ability to manage your financial future. As you continue to learn, set goals, and take control of your finances, you not only change your own life but also inspire others to begin their own journeys.

Remember, financial independence is more than a destination—it is a lifelong practice that evolves with you. Stay curious, stay empowered, and continue embracing your power over your financial destiny.

15. LEADERSHIP AND EMPOWERMENT

Leadership and Empowerment

Financial empowerment extends far beyond mere wealth; it's about autonomy, security, and the freedom to shape one's future. As a woman, my path to financial empowerment has been marked by both unique challenges and powerful victories. In this chapter, I will share my perspective on why financial empowerment is essential, the hurdles I've encountered, and the strategies I've used to achieve independence. My story is one of resilience, determination, and a firm belief that every woman has the power to take control of her financial destiny.

The Importance of Financial Empowerment

For women, financial empowerment is not simply about managing money. It's about breaking free from societal constraints and paving the way for self-determination. Here are some of the distinct challenges I've faced along the way:

1. **Gender Wage Gap**: The persistent wage gap between men and women has limited my earnings and financial growth. It serves as a constant reminder that financial equality is still a work in progress.
2. **Cultural Norms**: Societal expectations often influence our financial choices, at times discouraging women from pursuing financial independence.
3. **Balancing Multiple Roles**: Juggling career, family, and personal commitments can make it difficult to prioritize financial planning.
4. **Lack of Financial Education**: The absence of accessible financial education has left me navigating complex

financial systems with limited guidance, leading to missed opportunities.

5. **Fear of Financial Independence**: The fear of disrupting relationships or social standing by asserting financial independence has held me back at times.

Strategies for Financial Empowerment

My journey toward financial empowerment has been transformative, shaped by strategies that have allowed me to take control of my financial destiny:

1. **Continuous Financial Education**: I am committed to learning about money management, investments, and financial planning. This knowledge became the foundation for making informed decisions.
2. **Goal Setting**: Establishing clear financial goals provided direction. Whether it was saving for retirement, paying off debt, or investing, having defined objectives kept me focused and motivated.
3. **Budgeting and Expense Management**: Budgeting has been essential in tracking my spending, reducing unnecessary expenses, and allocating funds wisely.
4. **Investment Acumen**: Gaining a deeper understanding of investment options enabled me to grow my wealth and secure my future.
5. **Negotiation Skills**: Honing negotiation skills was key to advocating for fair compensation and closing the wage gap. This empowered me to advance in my career.
6. **Embracing Financial Independence**: Celebrating financial independence has been my greatest victory, offering personal empowerment and control over my future.

Overcoming Common Challenges

Despite the obstacles, I learned to face these challenges head-on:

1. **Gender Wage Gap**: Through financial literacy and assertiveness, I've navigated this gap by advocating for fair pay and seeking opportunities that match my skills.
2. **Cultural Norms**: I learned to challenge societal expectations, making choices that aligned with my values and goals, even when they were unconventional.
3. **Balancing Multiple Roles**: By prioritizing financial well-being, I made time for financial planning amidst other responsibilities, ensuring that I wasn't neglecting my future.
4. **Financial Education**: I sought out resources and mentors to fill the knowledge gap, which reduced my financial stress and opened new doors.
5. **Fear of Independence**: I confronted the fear that financial independence might strain relationships, realizing that true empowerment often involves stepping outside of comfort zones.

Triumphs Along the Way

Each challenge has led to personal triumphs, reinforcing my belief in the transformative power of financial empowerment:

- **Financial Literacy**: With knowledge came empowerment. Financial education has helped me make smarter decisions, achieve my goals, and narrow the wage gap.
- **Investment Savvy**: Learning about investments has been crucial in building wealth and securing my financial future.

- **<u>Negotiation</u>**: Advocating for myself in financial matters has advanced my career and brought fair compensation.
- **<u>Celebrating Independence</u>**: Embracing my financial independence has been the ultimate reward, as it symbolizes freedom and control over my own life.

<u>Practical Tips and Resources</u>

1. **<u>Tools and Resources</u>**: To further your financial journey, consider exploring resources like *The Total Money Makeover* by Dave Ramsey, or financial apps such as Mint and YNAB (You Need A Budget). These tools can offer valuable insights and help manage finances effectively.
2. **<u>Actionable Steps</u>**: Begin by creating a personal budget, setting short- and long-term financial goals, and starting an emergency fund. Regularly review and adjust these elements as your financial situation evolves.

Encouragement and Motivation

1. **<u>Inspirational Quotes</u>: "The best way to predict your future is to create it."** — Peter Drucker. Let this quote remind you of the power you have to shape your financial destiny.
2. **<u>Words of Encouragement</u>**: Remember, every step you take towards financial independence is a victory. Even small progress is progress. Stay persistent and believe in your ability to overcome obstacles.

Interactive Components

• Self-Assessment Exercises:

- How would you assess your current financial situation? Are you clear on your financial goals?
- What areas of your financial management could use improvement? How might you address these areas?

• Personal Reflection Prompts:

- Reflect on a financial challenge you've faced. What strategies did you use to overcome it? What did you learn from the experience?
- Consider your biggest financial triumph. How did this success impact your confidence and future goals?

• Actionable Steps:

- What steps can you take today to begin or improve your financial planning? Consider creating or updating your budget and setting new financial goals.
- How can you incorporate continuous financial education into your routine? Explore resources or courses that align with your financial interests.

Future Trends and Outlook

1. **Emerging Trends**: Keep an eye on emerging trends such as digital currencies and sustainable investments. These can offer new opportunities for financial growth and impact.
2. **Evolving Strategies**: As financial tools and strategies evolve, stay informed about innovations in personal finance to continue optimizing your financial planning.

Community and Support

1. **Building a Support Network**: Connect with financial support groups or communities, either online or locally. Engaging with others who share your goals can provide encouragement and valuable insights.
2. **Mentorship and Advocacy**: Seek out mentors who can guide you in your financial journey, and consider becoming an advocate for financial education in your community to support others on their paths.

Celebrating the Journey

My journey toward financial empowerment has been a testament to my resilience and ability to rise above challenges. I celebrate the countless women who, like me, have faced these hurdles and emerged stronger. Together, we are shaping a future where financial independence is within reach for every woman.

Financial empowerment is not just about achieving personal success—it's about creating opportunities and positively impacting the lives of others. Our journeys are sources of inspiration, showing future generations that with persistence and determination, financial independence is possible for all.

The path to financial empowerment is ongoing, but every step forward is a victory, not just for ourselves, but for women everywhere. Let's continue to support one another on this journey, empowering ourselves and future generations to take control of their financial destinies.

As we reach the end of this chapter on leadership and financial empowerment, it's essential to reflect on the transformative power of financial independence and the profound impact it can have on your life. Financial empowerment is not merely about accumulating wealth—it's about reclaiming your autonomy, securing your future, and creating a life defined by choice and freedom.

Key Takeaways:

1. **Significance of Financial Empowerment**: Financial empowerment means breaking free from historical constraints and societal expectations. It's about claiming your right to financial security and control.

2. **Challenges Faced**: The journey towards financial empowerment involves overcoming obstacles such as the gender wage gap, cultural norms, balancing multiple roles, lack of financial education, and the fear of independence. Each challenge presents an opportunity for growth and resilience.

3. **Strategies for Success**: Embrace continuous financial education, set clear goals, develop budgeting skills, become investment-savvy, and hone your negotiation skills. Each strategy is a tool to help you navigate your financial journey and achieve independence.

4. **Triumphs and Celebrations**: Every challenge overcome and every victory achieved is a testament to your strength and determination. Celebrating these milestones reinforces your progress and empowers you to continue striving for greater achievements.

5. **Practical Tips and Resources**: Utilize tools and resources such as financial books, apps, and actionable steps to guide your financial planning. Regularly reviewing and adapting these elements will keep you on track toward your goals.

6. **Encouragement and Reflection**: Stay motivated by reflecting on your financial journey, acknowledging your successes, and setting new goals. Remember that every small step forward is a significant achievement.

7. **Community and Support**: Engage with financial support networks, seek mentorship, and become an advocate for financial education. Building a supportive

community can provide invaluable encouragement and insight.

Encouragement for Your Journey:

Your journey toward financial empowerment is ongoing and evolving. Embrace this process with confidence, knowing that each challenge faced, and each triumph celebrated contributes to your overall growth. As you continue to explore your financial potential, remember that the path to financial independence is as much about self-discovery as it is about managing money.

Allow your journey to inspire and guide you toward new heights. Celebrate every victory, learn from every setback, and remain steadfast in your commitment to taking control of your financial destiny. Your resilience and determination are powerful tools that will lead you to greater autonomy, security, and fulfillment.

Keep moving forward with courage and clarity. The path to financial empowerment is a lifelong adventure, and with each step, you are not only shaping your own future but also paving the way for others to follow. Embrace the journey, trust in your abilities, and continue to build a future where you can live on your terms.

Your financial journey is a testament to your strength, and every woman's story of empowerment adds to the collective force for change. Let this chapter be a catalyst for your ongoing quest for financial independence and self-discovery. The road ahead is filled with possibilities, and you have the power to navigate it with confidence and grace.

16. TURNING PASSION INTO PURPOSE

Turning Passion into Purpose

Turning passion into purpose is a transformative journey that allows us to channel our deepest desires and interests into a meaningful mission. For women, this process involves navigating unique challenges and seizing opportunities to align passion with purpose, ultimately creating a legacy of change. In this chapter, I will share insights on the significance of this alignment, the obstacles encountered, and the strategies employed to turn dreams into a purpose-driven reality. This journey is not just about self-discovery but about leaving a lasting impact and empowering others to embark on their paths.

The Significance of Turning Passion into Purpose

Aligning our passion with purpose extends beyond merely following our hearts; it involves making a positive impact. Women, with our inherent empathy, compassion, and deep understanding of community needs, possess a unique perspective on how to transform our passions into a force for good. This alignment fosters not only personal fulfillment but also contributes to broader societal change.

Unique Challenges and Opportunities

1. **Balancing Multiple Roles**: Women often juggle various roles—caregiving, careers, and community involvement. Finding time and energy to pursue passions amidst these responsibilities can be challenging.

- How do you manage to balance your roles while nurturing your passion?

- What strategies or tools have you found effective in managing your time and energy?

2. **Cultural Norms**: Cultural expectations can sometimes dissuade us from pursuing unconventional paths. These norms can stifle individuality and creativity.

   - How have cultural expectations influenced your journey?
   - What steps have you taken to challenge or overcome these cultural norms?

3. **Lack of Female Representation**: In many fields, the underrepresentation of women poses a challenge. Breaking into male-dominated spaces requires resilience and determination.

   - Have you encountered this barrier, and if so, how have you navigated it?
   - What support or resources have helped you in overcoming the lack of representation?

4. **Fear of Failure**: The fear of failure, along with concerns about judgment and criticism, can be particularly daunting.

   - How do you overcome this fear to keep pursuing your passions?
   - Can you share an example of how facing your fear of failure led to growth or success?

Strategies for Turning Passion into Purpose

1. Self-Discovery: Discovering your true passions involves exploring your interests, values, and strengths. This self-awareness is crucial for aligning passion with purpose.

- What methods have you used for self-discovery?
- How has self-discovery helped you clarify and pursue your purpose?

2. Goal Setting: Clear, purpose-driven goals provide direction and motivation. Setting and regularly reviewing these goals can help in maintaining focus.

- What strategies do you use to set and achieve your goals?
- How do you ensure that your goals remain aligned with your evolving passions?

3. Network and Support: Building a supportive network of like-minded individuals is essential. Mentors, peers, and communities can offer valuable guidance and encouragement.

- Who has been instrumental in your journey, and how has their support helped?
- What steps have you taken to build and nurture your network?

4. Resilience: Developing resilience to face setbacks and challenges is key. Embracing failure as a learning opportunity can turn obstacles into steppingstones.

- How do you cultivate resilience in your pursuit of purpose?
- Can you share a specific challenge you faced and how you overcame it with resilience?

5. <u>Advocacy:</u> Advocating for your passion and purpose helps drive change. Your unique voice can challenge stereotypes and push boundaries.

- In what ways do you advocate for yourself and your passions?
- How has advocacy played a role in advancing your purpose?

6. <u>Mentorship:</u> Engaging in mentorship, both as a mentor and mentee, enriches the journey. Guiding others and learning from their experiences fosters growth.

- How has mentorship played a role in your journey?
- What benefits have you experienced from being both a mentor and a mentee?

Personal Stories and Anecdotes

In this journey, real-life examples can provide inspiration and guidance. Consider the story of [Name], who transformed her passion for environmental conservation into a global initiative that has made a significant impact. Her journey from a small community project to a recognized global movement highlights the power of aligning passion with purpose.

Practical Exercises

1. **<u>Self-Discovery Exercise</u>**: Take some time to reflect on your interests, values, and strengths. Write down what excites you, what you are good at, and what values drive you. Use this reflection to identify potential passions that align with your sense of purpose.
2. **<u>Goal-Setting Worksheet</u>**: Create a worksheet with sections for short-term and long-term goals. Define specific, actionable steps for achieving these goals and set deadlines to keep yourself on track.

3. **Resilience Reflection**: Reflect on a past challenge and how you overcame it. Write about the lessons learned and how you can apply these lessons to your current journey.

Expert Insights

Incorporate wisdom from experts in the field. For instance, motivational speaker [Expert's Name] emphasizes the importance of resilience and perseverance in turning passion into purpose. Their insights can provide valuable perspectives and encouragement.

Action Plan

1. *Step 1:* Conduct a self-assessment to identify your passions, values, and strengths.
2. *Step 2:* Set specific, actionable goals that align with your identified passions.
3. *Step 3:* Build a support network by connecting with mentors, peers, and communities.
4. *Step 4:* Develop strategies to cultivate resilience and overcome setbacks.
5. *Step 5:* Engage in advocacy and mentorship to advance your purpose and support others.

Inspirational Quotes

- *"The only way to do great work is to love what you do."* — Steve Jobs
- "Passion is the fuel; purpose is the driver." — Unknown
- **"Your work is going to fill a large part of your life, and the only way to be truly satisfied is to do what you believe is great work."** — Steve Jobs

Additional Resources

Explore further with these resources:

- **<u>Books</u>**: *"Find Your Why"* **by Simon Sinek,** *"Daring Greatly"* by Brené Brown
- **<u>Online Courses</u>**: Look for courses on platforms like Coursera or Udemy focusing on goal setting, personal development, and leadership.
- **<u>Workshops</u>**: Attend workshops or webinars on passion-driven career paths and purpose-driven living.

Celebrating the Journey

The journey of turning passion into purpose is a testament to strength, resilience, and the capacity to effect change. It is not merely about pursuing personal interests but about creating a legacy that empowers and uplifts others.

- How do you celebrate your milestones and the impact you've made?
- What achievements are you most proud of in your journey so far?

Ongoing Process of Growth

Turning passion into purpose is an ongoing journey that requires continual nurturing and growth. Regularly revisiting your goals, staying connected to your passions, and engaging with your support network are essential.

- How do you maintain and evolve your sense of purpose?
- What practices or routines help you stay aligned with your passions?

The Ever-Present Significance of Purpose

Living a purpose-driven life transcends personal fulfillment; it is about making a lasting impact. This journey reflects the enduring significance of aligning passion with purpose and using it to drive meaningful change.

- As you reflect on your path, what lasting impact do you hope to make?
- How do you envision your purpose evolving?

A Call to Action

This chapter serves as a call to action for women to transform their passions into a powerful purpose. It is an invitation to break through barriers, create lasting change, and inspire others to embark on their purpose-driven journeys.

- How will you use your passion to create a legacy of empowerment and positive impact?
- What steps will you take to inspire and support others in their journey of turning passion into purpose?

By reflecting on these questions and strategies, we can collectively turn our passions into purposeful action, creating a ripple effect of change and empowerment that resonates through generations.

Turning passion into purpose is not a one-time achievement but a continuous journey of growth, discovery, and impact. As we navigate this path, we confront challenges, seize opportunities, and transform our deepest desires into meaningful missions that resonate far beyond ourselves. This chapter has explored the profound significance of aligning passion with purpose, identified the unique obstacles women face, and offered practical strategies to overcome these barriers and build a legacy of empowerment.

Summary

In this chapter, we have delved into the essence of turning passion into purpose and the unique challenges and opportunities that come with this journey for women. We discussed the importance of balancing multiple roles, overcoming cultural norms, addressing the lack of female representation, and managing the fear of failure. Through the strategies of self-discovery, goal setting, building a supportive network, fostering resilience, advocacy, and mentorship, we can effectively transform our passions into a driving force for change.

Key Takeaways:

1. **Significance of Purpose**: Aligning passion with purpose creates a powerful impact, allowing us to make a positive difference in the world while achieving personal fulfillment.
2. **Challenges**: Women often face unique challenges such as balancing multiple roles, cultural expectations, and a lack of representation in certain fields. Understanding and addressing these challenges is crucial for moving forward.
3. **Strategies for Success**: Engaging in self-discovery, setting clear goals, building a supportive network, cultivating resilience, advocating for your passions, and participating in mentorship are essential strategies for turning passion into purpose.
4. **Celebrating Milestones**: Recognizing and celebrating your achievements along the way not only reinforces your journey but also motivates continued growth and impact.
5. **Ongoing Growth**: Turning passion into purpose is an ongoing process that requires regular reflection, adaptation, and nurturing. Staying connected to your

passions and evolving your goals ensures that your purpose remains relevant and impactful.

Encouragement

As you continue your journey of self-discovery and purpose, remember that this path is as much about the journey itself as it is about the destination. Embrace the challenges, celebrate your progress, and stay committed to your goals. Your unique passions and purpose have the potential to create a legacy of positive change and empowerment.

Let your passion be the guiding light that propels you forward, and let your purpose be the foundation upon which you build a meaningful and impactful life. The world needs your voice, your vision, and your contributions. Keep moving forward with confidence, knowing that each step you take brings you closer to turning your dreams into a powerful, purpose-driven reality.

Embrace this journey with courage and resilience and continue to inspire and uplift others along the way. Your path is a testament to the strength and determination that women possess, and it is a call to action for all who seek to transform their passions into a legacy of change.

17. RESILIENCE IN THE FACE OF SETBACKS

Resilience in the Face of Setbacks

Resilience is the cornerstone of a woman's journey — a path marked by setbacks, challenges, and triumphs. In this chapter, I will explore the profound significance of resilience, share personal experiences, and outline strategies for turning setbacks into steppingstones towards success. I aim to inspire and support others as they navigate their journeys of resilience.

The Significance of Resilience

Resilience is more than just bouncing back from adversity; it's about emerging stronger, wiser, and more empowered. As women, our unique challenges make resilience an essential quality. We embody strength, and our capacity to persevere in the face of obstacles is a testament to the power of resilience.

Unique Challenges and Opportunities

1. **Gender Bias**: Women often face additional barriers due to persistent gender bias, which can impact career opportunities and personal aspirations.
2. **Balancing Multiple Roles**: Juggling responsibilities as caregivers, professionals, and partners can be overwhelming, impacting our ability to remain resilient.
3. **Societal Expectations**: The pressure to conform to societal norms can be stifling, making it challenging to bounce back from setbacks.
4. **Imposter Syndrome**: Many women struggle with imposter syndrome, which can undermine confidence and resilience.

Strategies for Building Resilience

1. **Self-awareness**: Developing self-awareness is fundamental. Understanding your emotions and reactions helps in managing setbacks effectively.
2. **Positive Mindset**: A positive mindset allows you to view setbacks as growth opportunities. Focusing on what you can learn from adversity strengthens resilience.
3. **Support System**: Building a strong network of friends, family, and mentors provides crucial emotional support and guidance during tough times.
4. **Adaptability**: Being flexible and open to change is vital. Adaptability enables you to handle challenges and bounce back more effectively.
5. **Self-Compassion**: Practicing self-compassion helps maintain self-esteem and resilience. Treat yourself with kindness during setbacks.
6. **Goal Setting**: Clear, purpose-driven goals provide direction and motivation, helping you continue progressing despite obstacles.

Celebrating Resilience

Resilience is not just about overcoming challenges; it's about thriving because of them. My journey is a testament to the strength, adaptability, and determination that women possess. Each setback has been a steppingstone to greater empowerment and success.

Personal Stories of Resilience

One significant moment in my journey involved a major career setback. I was overlooked for a promotion I had worked tirelessly towards. The disappointment was immense, but I chose to practice the strategies I advocate. I recognized my feelings, reframed the setback as an opportunity for growth, and leaned on my support system for guidance. Adaptability helped me refine my approach, while self-compassion preserved my self-esteem. Ultimately, I secured the promotion, proving that resilience is not just a quality but a practical set of strategies.

Interaction Questions

1. **Reflecting on Challenges**: What unique challenges have you faced in your journey? How have these challenges shaped your understanding of resilience?
2. **Personal Strategies**: What strategies have you used to build resilience in your own life? Which ones have been most effective for you?
3. **Support Systems**: Who has been a part of your support system during challenging times? How has their support impacted your resilience?
4. **Overcoming Setbacks**: Can you share a personal story of a setback you faced and how you turned it into an opportunity for growth?

The Ever-Present Significance of Resilience

Resilience remains central to navigating life's complexities. It's about not just bouncing back but emerging stronger and more empowered. Resilience is a beacon of strength, determination, and adaptability.

A Journey of Personal Growth

My journey through resilience has catalyzed profound personal growth. I've learned the value of adaptability, determination, and a positive mindset. This journey has expanded my horizons and bolstered my confidence in facing challenges.

Celebrating the Legacy

My journey is a call to action for all women to turn challenges into opportunities for growth. Embracing resilience as a tool for personal development allows us to break barriers, challenge norms, and inspire others. Resilience is not just about overcoming adversity; it's about thriving because of it. This legacy of resilience empowers us to build a future where strength and perseverance are celebrated.

Role Models of Resilience

Highlight stories of notable women who exemplify resilience. This could include historical figures, contemporary leaders, or even lesser-known individuals who have overcome significant obstacles. Sharing these stories can provide inspiration and practical examples of resilience in action.

Interactive Exercises

1. **Resilience Reflection Worksheet**: Include a worksheet or set of prompts that readers can use to reflect on their resilience journey. For example, they might list past setbacks, the strategies they used to overcome them, and the lessons learned.
2. **Resilience Action Plan**: Provide a template for readers to create their resilience action plan. This could include setting specific goals, identifying potential setbacks, and outlining strategies for overcoming them.

Expert Insights

Incorporate quotes or insights from psychologists, coaches, or other experts on resilience. This adds credibility and provides readers with professional perspectives on building resilience.

Practical Tips and Resources

1. **Books and Articles**: Recommend books, articles, or podcasts that focus on resilience and personal development.
2. **Support Networks**: Provide information on how to find or build a support network, including resources for finding mentors, joining support groups, or accessing professional guidance.

Enhanced Interaction Questions

1. **Learning from Role Models**: Who are some role models you look up to for their resilience? How have their stories influenced your approach to handling setbacks?
2. **Personal Resilience Strategies**: What new strategies or techniques would you like to try to enhance your resilience? How do you plan to implement them?
3. **Impact of Resilience on Others**: How has your resilience influenced those around you? Share an example of how your ability to bounce back from challenges has impacted your family, friends, or colleagues.
4. **Future Resilience Goals**: What are your long-term goals for building resilience? How will you measure your progress and stay motivated?

Resilience is a powerful, transformative quality that defines our ability to navigate the ups and downs of life. This chapter has explored the profound significance of resilience, the unique challenges women face, and the practical strategies to build and nurture this vital trait. We've delved into personal stories of triumph, highlighted notable role models, and shared actionable steps to turn setbacks into opportunities for growth.

<u>Key Takeaways:</u>

1. **<u>Embrace Resilience as Strength</u>**: Resilience is not just about bouncing back from adversity; it's about emerging stronger and more empowered. It's a testament to the strength and adaptability that women possess.

2. **<u>Recognize Unique Challenges</u>**: Understand and acknowledge the unique challenges that women face, including gender bias, balancing multiple roles, societal expectations, and imposter syndrome. Each challenge is an opportunity to build resilience.

3. **<u>Employ Effective Strategies</u>**: Use strategies such as self-awareness, maintaining a positive mindset, building a support system, embracing adaptability, practicing self-compassion, and setting clear goals to enhance your resilience.

4. **<u>Celebrate Your Journey</u>**: Reflect on your personal stories of overcoming setbacks and celebrate your resilience. Recognize the strength, adaptability, and determination that have shaped your journey.

5. **<u>Learn from Others</u>**: Draw inspiration from role models who exemplify resilience. Their stories can provide valuable insights and motivation for your journey.

6. **<u>Continue Your Journey</u>**: Building resilience is an ongoing process. Use the interactive exercises, expert insights, and practical tips shared in this chapter to continue developing and nurturing your resilience.

As you move forward on your path of self-discovery, remember that resilience is a continuous journey of growth and empowerment. Each challenge you face is a steppingstone towards greater strength and understanding. Embrace your setbacks as opportunities to learn, adapt, and thrive. Your journey is not just about overcoming adversity; it is about shaping a legacy of resilience that empowers you and inspires those around you.

Encouragement for the Journey Ahead:

Keep pushing forward with the knowledge that resilience is a powerful tool for personal growth and success. Your ability to adapt, persevere, and emerge stronger is a testament to your inner strength and determination. Continue to embrace resilience, and let it guide you through life's challenges. Celebrate your progress, learn from each experience, and inspire others with your journey.

You have the power to turn setbacks into steppingstones and to build a legacy of resilience that will carry you through the many adventures and challenges that lie ahead. Embrace this journey with courage, confidence, and unwavering determination. Your story of resilience is one of empowerment and inspiration—one that will continue to evolve and inspire for years to come.

18. INSPIRING AND UPLIFTING

Inspiring and Uplifting

As women, we possess an incredible and unique power to inspire and uplift each other. In this chapter, I will share my perspective on the profound importance of empowering our fellow women, the challenges we may face, and the strategies I have embraced to become a source of inspiration and strength for others. My journey reflects the belief that, together, we can create a powerful collective force of empowerment that transcends individual achievements. My mission is not just personal; it's a call to support others as they embark on their paths to inspire and uplift.

The Power of Inspiring and Uplifting Women

Supporting and uplifting women goes beyond individual growth—it builds a community of strength. When we come together to uplift each other, we create a ripple effect that extends far beyond our successes, generating empowerment for future generations.

Challenges and Opportunities

1. **Overcoming Competitiveness**: Society often fosters competition among women. To truly inspire and uplift, we must rise above this competitiveness and work in solidarity.
2. **Self-Doubt and Imposter Syndrome**: Many women experience self-doubt and imposter syndrome, hindering their ability to reach their full potential. Supporting one another through these challenges becomes essential.

3. **<u>Balancing Multiple Roles</u>**: Women often juggle various roles—professionals, caregivers, partners—which can make it difficult to find time and energy to support others. But it's in this balancing act that we also find the strength to uplift.

4. **<u>Breaking Cultural Norms</u>**: Societal norms and expectations can influence the way women interact. Challenging these norms is crucial in creating an atmosphere where uplifting others is the norm, not the exception.

<u>Long-Term Impact of Uplifting Women</u>

When women come together to inspire and uplift each other, the effects ripple out far beyond the individual or the community—it reshapes society. Studies have shown that communities and organizations with empowered women tend to be more inclusive, innovative, and prosperous. By championing each other, we create a future where women have greater access to leadership roles, economic opportunities, and influence in policymaking.

Empowered women also inspire the next generation of young girls to aim higher. By modeling collaboration and support, we teach the future generation that they don't need to compete to succeed; instead, they can rise together, creating a culture where collaboration and empowerment are the norm.

<u>Real-Life Examples of Women Empowering Women</u>

1. <u>Sheryl Sandberg & Lean in Circles</u>: The COO of Facebook, Sheryl Sandberg, launched Lean In Circles, a global network that encourages women to support each other professionally and personally. This initiative shows the power of creating spaces where women uplift one another.

2. <u>Oprah Winfrey's Mentorship and Philanthropy</u>: Oprah Winfrey's legacy is built on mentorship and empowerment. Through her Leadership Academy for Girls and countless mentorship programs, she uplifts women and girls to reach for their dreams.

3. <u>The #MeToo Movement</u>: This global movement started when women came together to amplify each other's voices and break the silence around sexual harassment. The collective strength of women sharing their stories inspired legislative changes, corporate reforms, and broader societal shifts.

<u>Expanding Your Role in Uplifting Others</u>

In your journey to inspire and uplift others, it's important to continually reflect on your role in the movement. Are you actively seeking out opportunities to mentor, amplify, and empower other women in your community or workplace? Consider how you can step further into this role and create an even larger impact.

<u>Strategies for Inspiring and Uplifting Women</u>

1. **<u>Mentorship</u>:** Being a mentor allows us to share our experiences and provide guidance. Equally important is seeking out mentors who inspire and challenge us to grow.
2. **<u>Networking</u>:** Building a network of like-minded women who share your goals and values creates a foundation for mutual support and inspiration.
3. **<u>Lifting as You Climb</u>:** Embrace the philosophy that your success is not solitary. As you rise, bring others with you—celebrate their victories as if they were your own.
4. **<u>Collaboration Over Competition</u>:** Replace competition with collaboration. When women work together

towards shared goals, they not only uplift one another but also create environments where everyone thrives.

5. **Building Confidence**: Encourage other women to develop self-confidence. Empower them to overcome self-doubt and embrace their full potential.
6. **Amplifying Voices**: Elevate the voices of other women. Share their stories, ideas, and achievements, and make space for them to shine.

Triumphs and Milestones

Throughout my journey, I have encountered challenges, but I have also experienced triumphs that fuel my commitment to uplifting others:

- **Mentorship** has been one of my greatest triumphs, providing guidance and inspiration to other women while enriching my own journey.
- **Networking** has given me access to a powerful support system of like-minded women, which has strengthened my resolve and offered opportunities for mutual growth.
- **Lifting as You Climb** has instilled a sense of unity and shared purpose in everything I do, reminding me that success is not singular.
- **Collaboration** has opened doors to collective achievement, and I have seen firsthand how much stronger we are when we work together.

Celebrating Our Collective Journey

This journey is not solely about individual achievement but about building a legacy of empowerment that reaches across generations. We are crafting a future where women are not just personally successful, but are collectively shaping the world in meaningful, lasting ways.

As I continue my path of inspiring and uplifting women, I am reminded of the profound power that comes from unity and collaboration. We are an unstoppable force, creating an enduring legacy of empowerment that breaks through barriers, challenges societal norms, and fosters an environment where every woman can thrive.

Interactive Reflection Questions

1. **In what ways can you inspire and uplift the women around you?** Consider your own experiences and strengths—how can they be shared with others?
2. **Have you ever experienced competitiveness with another woman?** How did it affect you, and how might collaboration have created a different outcome?
3. **What are some strategies you can implement to overcome self-doubt and imposter syndrome?** How can you help others do the same?
4. **Think about a time when someone amplified your voice.** How did that make you feel, and how can you pay it forward by doing the same for another woman today?

Our journey of inspiring and uplifting women is not just a personal endeavor; it's a collective mission. By embracing the power of mentorship, collaboration, and empowerment, we become a force for change that can redefine the future. Together, we are stronger, bolder, and more unstoppable than we ever could be alone. Let's celebrate and continue to inspire the next generation of women, leaving behind a legacy of strength, unity, and empowerment.

Embracing the Power of Uplifting One Another

As women, we are uniquely equipped to inspire and uplift each other, and in doing so, we create a world where collective strength far surpasses individual success. This chapter has explored the significance of building a community of empowered women, the challenges we face in overcoming competitiveness and self-doubt, and the strategies that help us turn competition into collaboration. By mentoring, networking, and amplifying each other's voices, we become a unified force that changes not only our own lives but the world around us.

The journey of inspiring and uplifting other women is not without its obstacles, but the triumphs are profound. Together, we can overcome societal norms, break free from limitations, and set an example for future generations. Let this chapter serve as a reminder that, as we lift others, we elevate ourselves, and in doing so, we leave behind a legacy of strength, unity, and empowerment.

Key Takeaways

1. **Inspiring and uplifting other women** is not just about personal success—it builds a community of strength, empowerment, and unity that creates a lasting impact on society.
2. **Challenges** such as competitiveness, self-doubt, and cultural norms are real, but by working together, we can overcome these obstacles.
3. **Mentorship and networking** provide critical pathways for empowerment, allowing women to share knowledge, offer guidance, and build supportive connections.
4. **Collaboration over competition** creates environments where women thrive collectively, sharing in one another's successes.
5. **Lifting as you climb** is a philosophy that ensures the success of one woman becomes the success of many, and it builds a powerful foundation for future generations.

6. <u>**Amplifying voices**</u> and building **self-confidence** in other women ensures that the legacy of empowerment continues to grow, with every woman supporting the next.

<u>Encouragement for Continued Growth</u>

As you reflect on this chapter, consider how you can continue your journey of self-discovery and growth. How can you become an even stronger source of inspiration and support for the women around you? Whether it's through mentoring, advocating for equality, or simply offering encouragement, every act of upliftment contributes to the greater legacy of women's empowerment.

I encourage you to seek out opportunities to empower others, and in doing so, you will find that your own journey of self-discovery deepens. The ripple effect of your actions will be felt not just by the women in your immediate circle, but by future generations. Together, we can transform communities, inspire new possibilities, and shape a world where women are not just successful but truly unstoppable.

19. CELEBRATING YOUR VICTORIES

Celebrating Your Victories

As an unstoppable woman, every victory — whether monumental or modest — reflects the strength, resilience, and determination that drives our journey. In this chapter, I will share the significance of celebrating our achievements, the challenges we face in doing so, and strategies I've embraced to savor victories to the fullest. My journey isn't solely about the pursuit of success; it's about embracing the joy of every triumph and inspiring others to do the same.

The Significance of Celebrating Victories

Celebrating victories goes beyond merely acknowledging what we've achieved; it's about recognizing the immense effort, perseverance, and inner strength it took to get there. As unstoppable women, we navigate obstacles, break barriers, and overcome doubts. Each celebration is a deserved moment to honor that journey and refuel our spirits for the road ahead.

But celebrating victories is not just personal — it's transformational. When we take time to honor our success, we're not only validating ourselves but also modeling the importance of joy in the journey. This act of self-affirmation builds confidence and sets an example for other women who may struggle to celebrate their own wins.

Personal Story: My Journey to Celebration

I remember a time when I found it difficult to celebrate my successes. I had achieved a significant career milestone — one I had worked tirelessly for. But instead of basking in the joy, I felt guilty, worried about coming across as arrogant or self-centered. I downplayed my accomplishment, barely mentioning it to those around me.

It wasn't until a close friend sat me down and said, "Why are you hiding your light?" that I realized how much I had diminished my own success. She helped me understand that my victory wasn't just about me — it was about the perseverance and strength that got me there. She also reminded me that celebrating would inspire others to push through their own struggles. That conversation changed my perspective. From that moment forward, I began to embrace my wins with grace, humility, and joy, and it has since fueled my continued growth.

Interactive question:
Have you ever downplayed a victory? How did that make you feel? How might celebrating it have changed your outlook?

Unique Challenges and Opportunities:

1. **Balancing Humility and Pride:** As women, societal pressures may compel us to downplay our achievements for fear of being perceived as boastful. However, pride in our accomplishments is necessary for growth. The challenge lies in confidently owning our success while maintaining humility.
2. **Imposter Syndrome:** Even in moments of triumph, feelings of doubt can creep in, causing us to question whether we truly deserve our success. Recognizing and overcoming these thoughts is key to fully embracing our victories.
3. **Finding Support and Validation:** It can be difficult to find people who fully understand the significance of our wins. Celebrating can feel isolating if those around us aren't able to appreciate the effort we've invested. Having a strong support system is essential for shared joy.

<u>Strategies for Celebrating Victories</u>

1. <u>**Self-Reflection:**</u> Take time to reflect on your journey—the obstacles you've overcome, the growth you've achieved, and the lessons learned. It's a powerful way to deeply appreciate the effort behind each victory.

   Interactive question:
   <u>*When was the last time you reflected on your achievements? How did it feel to acknowledge your progress?*</u>

2. <u>**Share with a Supportive Network:**</u> Surround yourself with people who understand the significance of your accomplishments. Sharing your triumphs with those who uplift you makes celebration richer and more meaningful.

   Interactive question:
   <u>*Who in your life truly understands and celebrates your achievements with you? How can you strengthen that connection?*</u>

3. <u>**Set New Goals:**</u> Every victory is a steppingstone to the next. Setting new goals not only keeps the momentum going but ensures that you continue growing and pushing yourself beyond your current limits.

4. <u>**Embrace Self-Compassion:**</u> Practice self-compassion by acknowledging that it's okay to take pride in your hard work. Celebrating yourself is not arrogance—it's an important part of recognizing the dedication and energy you've invested in your success.

5. <u>**Inspire Others:**</u> Use your victories to uplift others. Sharing your journey can empower those around you to celebrate their own wins, creating a ripple effect of joy and self-confidence.

Interactive question:
How can your victories inspire others around you? Can
you think of someone who might benefit from hearing
about your journey?

Rituals of Celebration

Incorporating personal rituals into your celebrations can deepen the experience and help reinforce the importance of each achievement. Whether it's writing about your win in a journal, taking a moment of stillness, or treating yourself to something meaningful, rituals turn celebrations into cherished memories.

- **Create Traditions:** Establish personal traditions to mark your victories. It could be as simple as lighting a candle or treating yourself to a favorite experience.

  Interactive question:
  What personal ritual can you create to honor your
  victories?

The Power of Gratitude

Gratitude amplifies the joy of celebration. By expressing appreciation for the people, opportunities, and even challenges that have shaped your journey, you foster a positive cycle of success and fulfillment.

- **Gratitude Journaling:** Take time to write down the things you are grateful for in connection with each victory. This practice grounds your achievements in a sense of abundance and helps you appreciate the full scope of your journey.

<u>Interactive question:</u>
<u>What are you grateful for in your latest victory? Who</u>
<u>or what helped you achieve it?</u>

<u>Celebrating with Others</u>

While personal reflection is vital, shared joy is often even more powerful. Invite others to celebrate with you, whether through small gatherings, virtual parties, or simply sharing your success on social media. This collective celebration builds connections and reinforces the importance of community support.

- **<u>Host a Victory Gathering:</u>** Bring together the people who supported you along your journey. Whether it's a simple coffee chat or a larger event, celebrating together deepens your connections and adds richness to the experience.

  <u>Interactive question:</u>
  <u>Who would you invite to your victory celebration?</u>
  <u>How can you thank them for their support?</u>

<u>Victory Vault</u>

Consider keeping a **"Victory Vault"** — a collection of mementos, notes, or memories from your successes. Whether it's a physical box, a digital folder, or a vision board, this vault will serve as a reminder of your unstoppable journey whenever you need encouragement.

<u>Interactive question:</u>
<u>What will you place in your Victory Vault to remind you of</u>
<u>your strength during challenging times?</u>

Embracing Setbacks as Part of the Celebration

Victories often follow setbacks. Learning to celebrate the resilience it took to overcome obstacles enhances the sweetness of success. Honor not only the win but also the journey that got you there.

- **Honor the Struggles:** Reflect on the challenges that shaped your success. Recognize that each setback contributed to your growth and made your victory even more meaningful.

  Interactive question:
  What setback did you overcome in your latest victory? How did it shape your journey?

Legacy of Collective Empowerment

Your celebration is part of a larger movement. By lifting yourself and others up, you contribute to a legacy that empowers future generations. Each time you celebrate a victory; you are helping to build a culture of unstoppable women who take pride in their achievements.

- **Passing the Torch:** Consider mentoring someone earlier in their journey. Celebrate their wins as you celebrate your own, continuing the cycle of empowerment.

  Interactive question:
  Who can you mentor and encourage in their own journey of victories?

Victory as a Catalyst for Growth

Celebrating victories is not just about marking the end of a challenge — it's about acknowledging the growth, resilience, and perseverance that got you there. Each success, big or small, deserves recognition because it reflects your strength and determination. In this chapter, we explored how celebration isn't a luxury but an essential part of the unstoppable woman's journey. By reflecting on our wins, sharing them with a supportive network, setting new goals, and inspiring others, we make victory a tool for continuous growth.

But the celebration doesn't end with a single triumph. It's an ongoing journey of self-discovery, where each achievement serves as a steppingstone toward greater heights. Embracing self-compassion, practicing gratitude, and creating rituals of celebration can turn your wins into lasting moments of empowerment. The challenges you've overcome are as much a part of your success as the result, and honoring that entire process enriches your life.

As you move forward, remember that your journey is unique and worth celebrating. Whether you're experiencing moments of joy, facing setbacks, or supporting others in their victories, each step is part of a larger story that you are writing. Continue to explore your strengths, embrace your growth, and celebrate every milestone—because in doing so, you not only uplift yourself but inspire others to rise alongside you.

Interactive question:
How will you turn victory into a way of life?

Key Takeaways:

1. **Celebrate Every Victory** – Acknowledge the strength, effort, and determination behind every success, no matter how small.

2. **<u>Reflect and Grow</u>** – Self-reflection deepens your appreciation for the journey and provides valuable insights for future growth.
3. **<u>Share the Joy</u>** – Surround yourself with supportive people who can celebrate your achievements with you, amplifying the joy.
4. **<u>Inspire Others</u>** – Use your victories as a source of inspiration and empowerment for those around you, creating a ripple effect of growth.
5. **<u>Keep Moving Forward</u>** – Set new goals and embrace challenges, using each victory as a steppingstone toward continued progress.

<u>Encouragement for the Journey Ahead</u>: Your journey of self-discovery and personal growth is ongoing. Every step forward is a chance to explore new possibilities, overcome fresh challenges, and continue building your legacy. Celebrate each milestone, learn from every setback, and keep pushing forward. Remember, you are unstoppable—and your victories, both past and future, are proof of that truth. Keep rising, keep discovering, and keep celebrating—you are capable of more than you ever imagined.

20. BECOMING UNSTOPPABLE

Becoming Unstoppable

In a world brimming with dreams, aspirations, and challenges, every woman holds the potential to become truly unstoppable. It's a transformative journey — one that goes beyond mere personal achievement. It is a quest for empowerment, breaking through barriers, and embracing the unique power we each possess. Through this chapter, I'll share my perspective on becoming unstoppable, the obstacles we face, and the strategies that can turn hurdles into steppingstones.

The Significance of Being Unstoppable

Becoming unstoppable is more than a personal triumph — it's about realizing your full potential and inspiring others to do the same. It's about breaking free from self-doubt, recognizing your worth, and embarking on a journey that not only empowers you but also uplifts others. This is how we break free from limitations and create ripples of change in the lives of others.

Unique Challenges and Opportunities

1. **Self-Doubt**: Self-doubt is often our first barrier. It's that voice in our heads telling us we aren't ready or worthy. But this adversary can be overcome by tapping into self-belief.
2. **Societal Expectations**: Society may impose restrictive roles, especially for women, shaping who we are "supposed" to be. Yet, the challenge is to rise above those expectations and define empowerment on our terms.

3. **<u>Balancing Multiple Roles</u>**: Whether as caregivers, professionals, or partners, we often juggle multiple roles. Finding time for self-growth amidst these responsibilities is tough, but necessary for becoming unstoppable.

<u>Strategies for Becoming Unstoppable</u>

1. **<u>Self-Discovery</u>**: Begin with understanding who you are at your core. Explore your values, strengths, and passions. When you know what drives you, empowerment naturally follows.
2. **<u>Setting Bold Goals</u>**: Purpose-driven, bold goals are your compass. Define them with clarity, and let them guide your actions and decisions.
3. **<u>Continuous Learning</u>**: Always be a student of life. Invest in your education and growth. Learning opens doors to new opportunities and fuels your drive.
4. **<u>Resilience</u>**: Cultivate resilience. Understand that setbacks are a natural part of progress. Each one is a chance to learn, adapt, and push forward.
5. **<u>Self-Care</u>**: You can't pour from an empty cup. Taking care of your mental, emotional, and physical well-being ensures you have the strength to pursue your goals.
6. **<u>Support System</u>**: Surround yourself with those who uplift you — mentors, friends, and a like-minded network that encourages you through the highs and lows.
7. **<u>Amplify Your Voice</u>**: Don't be afraid to share your story. Your journey has the power to inspire and encourage others. Speaking up for yourself and others can be transformative.
8. **<u>Empower Others</u>**: As you climb, reach back and support others on their path. This not only strengthens them but also reinforces your own empowerment.

A Story of Becoming Unstoppable: Sara Blakely

Sara Blakely, founder of Spanx, is a prime example of an unstoppable woman. She began her journey with an idea for footless pantyhose but faced countless rejections from manufacturers and investors. With a small budget, a dream, and relentless determination, she turned her vision into a billion-dollar business. Her story showcases how self-belief, resilience, and bold goals can lead to extraordinary achievements.

Sara often says, **"It was the failure along the way that built my resilience."** Her perseverance, despite obstacles, and her willingness to take risks have not only led to her personal success but have inspired women globally to pursue their dreams fearlessly.

Common Challenges We All Face

1. **Self-Doubt**: Like Sara Blakely, we all have moments where doubt creeps in. How often have you hesitated to take a first step because you weren't sure if you were enough?
2. **Societal Expectations**: Have you ever felt constrained by what society expects from you? Perhaps there's a passion you've suppressed because it doesn't fit a certain mold?
3. **Balancing Roles**: Many of us find it difficult to carve out time for our dreams while managing our responsibilities. How do you manage your time, and is there space for self-empowerment?

The Power of Mentorship

In every journey, mentorship plays a crucial role. Women who have become unstoppable often have had mentors who believed in them, offered guidance, and helped navigate through challenges. Becoming unstoppable also involves becoming a mentor yourself. Who has mentored you in your journey, and how have they influenced your path?

Interactive Question:

- Who is a mentor that has inspired you, and how can you offer similar guidance to someone on their journey?

Triumphs Over Challenges

1. **Self-Discovery:** Taking time to explore your passions and strengths is the foundation of empowerment. What have you discovered about yourself on your own journey?
2. **Bold Goals:** What bold, purpose-driven goals have you set for yourself? How have they shaped your decisions and actions?
3. **Resilience:** Share a moment when a setback became an opportunity for growth. How did that experience build your resilience?

Embracing Failure as a Catalyst for Growth

Failure is often seen as a setback, but for an unstoppable woman, it is a powerful learning tool. Each failure brings with it the gift of insight — helping us to pivot, adapt, and come back stronger. It's crucial to shift the mindset from fearing failure to embracing it as an opportunity.

Interactive Question:

- Reflect on a moment of failure. How did it serve as a steppingstone for your future successes? How has it shaped your resilience?

Your "Why": A Source of Motivation

At the heart of becoming unstoppable is understanding your "why." What drives you? What fuels your passion? Clarifying your purpose not only keeps you focused but also helps you push through difficult times.

Interactive Question:

- What is your **"why"?** When things get tough, how does your purpose keep you going?

Practical Exercises for Empowerment

Consider adding a few exercises to make the chapter more interactive:

- **Vision Board Exercise**: Encourage readers to create a vision board filled with their dreams, goals, and inspirations. This serves as a daily reminder of what they're working towards.
- **Journaling Prompt**: Have readers write down their current challenges and brainstorm ways they can overcome them using the strategies outlined in the chapter.
- **Goal-Setting Exercise**: Guide readers through a simple process of setting one bold, purpose-driven goal and mapping out the steps to achieve it. What's one step they can take today?

Unstoppable Women in History

Including stories of other unstoppable women throughout history—figures like Rosa Parks, Malala Yousafzai, or Ruth Bader Ginsburg—could offer additional inspiration. These women's courage and determination in the face of adversity can serve as powerful examples of what's possible.

Interactive Question:

- Who is a historical or contemporary woman who embodies unstoppable resilience to you? How can you draw from their strength?

Call to Action: Becoming a Movement

The journey of becoming unstoppable is one that can spark a movement. By encouraging others to embrace their potential, we create a community of empowered women who uplift each other. It's not just about personal empowerment—it's about fostering a collective force of women who break boundaries and reshape the world around them.

Interactive Question:

- How can you use your voice or platform to support and uplift other women? How will you contribute to this movement of empowerment?

Celebrating the Unstoppable Woman

As we journey towards becoming unstoppable, it's important to celebrate the progress we've made. Each victory, no matter how small, is a step forward. Becoming unstoppable is not just about personal success; it's about becoming a beacon for others. Our stories are powerful tools for change, inspiring other women to overcome doubt, societal limitations, and to reach for their full potential.

A Journey of Legacy and Growth

Becoming unstoppable isn't only about our personal growth—it's about leaving a legacy for future generations. When we overcome self-doubt and societal expectations, we pave the way for others to do the same. Our empowerment becomes a collective force, inspiring others to rise above limitations and create change.

Reflecting on Your Journey

- What challenges have you faced on your path to becoming unstoppable?
- What strategies have helped you overcome obstacles?
- How can your journey inspire others to embrace their own empowerment?

Together, we celebrate not only our achievements but the legacy we're building for future generations. Becoming unstoppable is a choice we make every day, and by lifting others as we climb, we create a ripple of change that impacts the world.

End with a Declaration of Unstoppability

Invite the reader to craft their own personal declaration of being unstoppable. This is a powerful way to conclude the chapter, leaving readers with a sense of ownership over their journey.

Example Declaration:
"I am unstoppable because I embrace my strength, overcome my doubts, and inspire others along the way. My journey is my own, and I move forward with purpose, resilience, and unwavering determination."

This could be a signature practice for readers as they close the chapter, empowering them to declare their commitment to becoming unstoppable in their own lives.

Embracing Your Journey to Becoming Unstoppable

As we reach the end of this chapter, it's clear that becoming unstoppable is a transformative journey — one that is rooted in self-discovery, resilience, and empowerment. It's about breaking through the barriers of self-doubt, societal expectations, and the pressures of balancing multiple roles. The key takeaways from this chapter emphasize that every woman possesses the potential to become unstoppable. The power lies within each of us to take ownership of our path and inspire others along the way.

We've explored how:

- **Self-discovery** lays the foundation for empowerment by helping you understand your values, strengths, and passions.
- **Setting bold goals** keeps you focused and purpose-driven, allowing you to navigate challenges with intention.
- **Continuous learning and resilience** are crucial to overcoming setbacks, transforming them into steppingstones on the path to success.
- **Self-care** and a strong **support system** are essential to maintaining the strength, energy, and motivation to keep going.
- **Amplifying your voice** and **empowering others** are not just acts of personal growth but of collective empowerment.

This journey is not just for your benefit — it's an invitation for every woman to embrace her potential, break free from societal constraints, and become a force of change for others. Becoming unstoppable is a continuous process of growth, courage, and learning. It is a legacy of empowerment that we create not only for ourselves but for generations to come.

Continue Your Journey

As you move forward, remember that this journey is uniquely yours. You have the strength to overcome any challenge, the resilience to rise after every setback, and the ability to inspire others through your story. Becoming unstoppable is not a destination but a lifelong commitment to self-growth and empowerment.

Take time to reflect on your **"why"**, celebrate your progress, and continue setting bold goals that align with your values. Embrace every lesson along the way and know that you are creating a powerful legacy of strength and inspiration for others.

The world needs your voice, your passion, and your unstoppable spirit. Keep pushing forward and always remember: You are unstoppable.

Interactive Question:

- What is the next step on your journey to becoming unstoppable? How can you act today to continue embracing your potential?

243